ASHTANGA
YOGA

Primary & Intermediate Series

Caroline Klebl, PhD

PUBLISHED BY
Source of Yoga

Ashtanga Yoga
Copyright © 2012 Caroline Klebl, PhD

Photographer: Carolyn Strover
Layout and Design: Anastasia Hockinson,
    Giyoung Park, Vilma Saldate, Bill Jonas
Editor: Emily Alp
Cover Design: Bill Jonas

Published by: Source of Yoga
Beverly Hills, CA

ISBN: 978-061556635-1

Dedicated to Sri K Pattabhi Jois

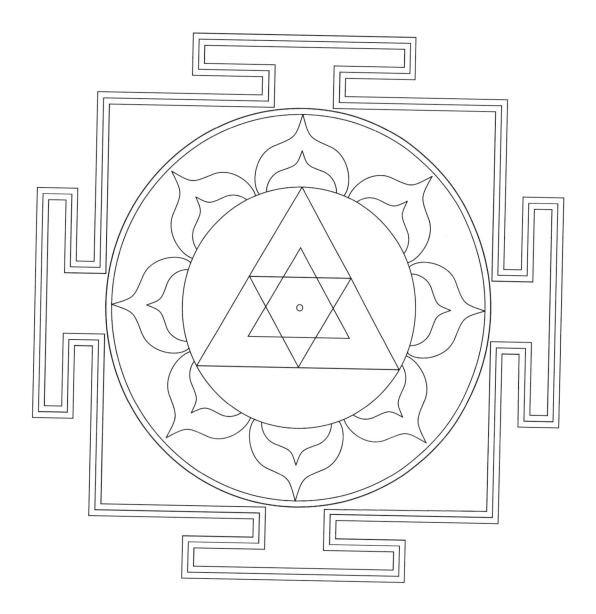

Ganesha Yantra

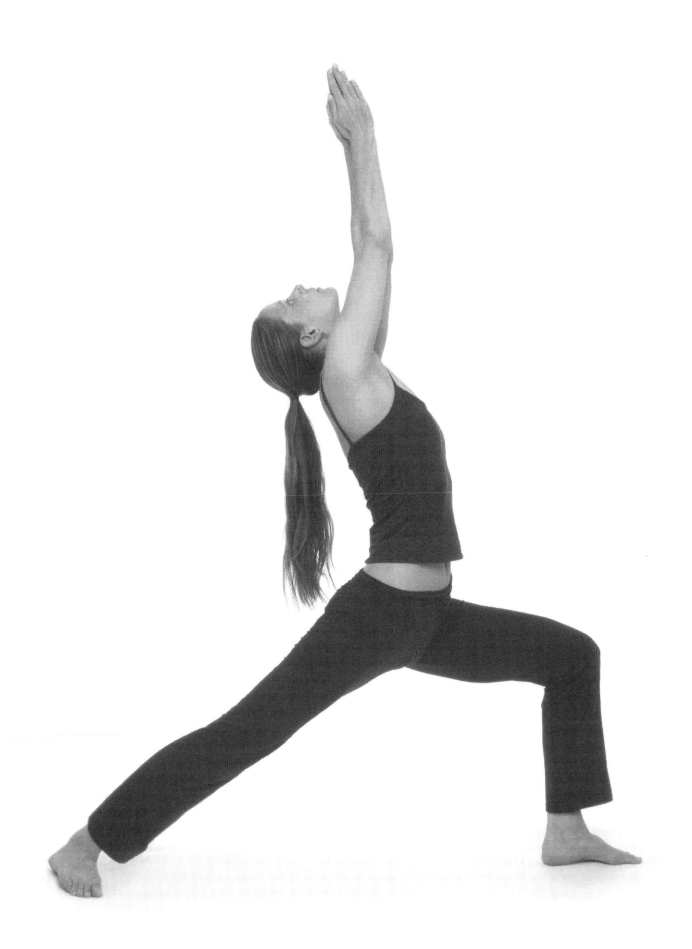

ASHTANGA
YOGA
Primary & Intermediate Series

CONTENTS

INTRODUCTION

Yoga is a 5000 year old tradition, which developed out of ancient Indian asceticism. *Yoga* is a Sanskrit word, which means union, but it is commonly known as spiritual discipline. Yoga is a tangible method of attaining to liberation from suffering and to the realization of supreme consciousness. There are six main types of Yoga mentioned in eastern philosophy: Karma Yoga (the Yoga of virtuous actions), Bhakti Yoga (the Yoga of love and devotion), Jnana Yoga (the Yoga of knowledge), Raja Yoga (meditation practice), Hatha Yoga (practice of yoga asanas [postures], pranayama [breathing techniques], mudras [sacred gestures] and kriyas [purification techniques]) and Tantra Yoga (recitation of mantra [sacred syllables], visualization of yantras [sacred diagrams], identification with deities and sexual practices).

Ashtanga Yoga, the eight steps of realization were described in the Yoga Sutras, a precise treatise on Yoga, which was compiled by the Sage Patanjali over 2000 years ago. The Yoga Sutras are divided into four padas (chapters or quarters): the Samadhi Pada, on consciousness; the Sadhana Pada describing various methods of yoga practice; the Vibhuti Pada, which enumerates the internal practices of concentration, meditation and absorption and the method of acquiring supernatural powers; and the Kaivalya Pada, which reveals the ultimate state of liberation.

The eight steps of yoga, which Ashtanga Yoga refers to, are defined in the Sadhana Pada, and individual steps are additionally referenced and described in detail throughout the entire Yoga Sutras text. Ashtanga is a Sanskrit term consisting of two words—"Ashta," translates as eight, and "Anga," translates as limbs, aspects or steps. Yoga is the unification of individual consciousness with supreme consciousness. The eight aspects of Yoga practice are yama (moral codes), niyama (applied disciplines), asana (posture), pranayama (breath-control), pratyahara (withdrawal of the sense organs), dharana (concentration), dhyana (meditation) and samadhi (absorption). Yoga is the unification of individual consciousness with supreme consciousness, and the eight steps of Ashtanga comprise structured and powerful practices for anyone willing to achieve this state.

The yamas are the moral codes, which ensure beneficial social interactions. They free the mind and life of a yoga practitioner from undesirable thoughts, feelings and circumstances resulting from immoral actions. The yamas include, ahimsa (non-violence), satya (truthfulness), asteya (non-theft), Brahmacharya (guided by Brahman or God) and aparighraha (non-hoarding).

The niyamas are those thoughts and actions that create a state of being that is conducive to yoga. The niyamas include saucha (cleanliness), santosha (contentment), tapas (heat from the practice of austerities), svadhyaya (chanting in reference to the study of supreme consciousness), Ishvara pranidhana (surrender to supreme consciousness or God).

The asana and pranayama practices are the gateway into the steps of Ashtanga Yoga. Asana practice is a tangible method for strengthening the body and eliminating disease. Pranayama practice awakens and purifies subtle energy channels underlying the physical form. The practice of asana and pranayama, clears impurities out of the body and induces a deeply meditative state, by which dysfunctional behavioral patterns are naturally abandoned.

In the Vibhuti Pada, the third chapter, of the Yoga Sutras, a separation of the eight limbs of Ashtanga Yoga into Bahiranga Sadhanas (external practices) and Antaranga Sadhanas (internal practices) is mentioned. The Bahiranga Sadhanas are comprised of yama, niyama, asana, pranayama and pratyahara. Pratyahara is the discipline of stopping the mind from making contact with objects through the sense organs.

INTRODUCTION

Pratyahara eliminates distractions, thereby enabling the practice of the subsequent Antaranga Sadhanas—dharana, dhyana and samadhi. Dharana is concentration in the form of binding of consciousness to one place or object. Dhyana, or meditation, is the exclusive extension of consciousness to this one place of object. And samadhi occurs when there is only awareness of this one place or object and there is no more awareness of one's self. Dharana, dhyana and samadhi taken together are called Samyama, which means control or restraint. By mastering Samyama the light of Prajna (intuition or insight) shines forth.

The world-renowned yoga Guru, Sri K Pattabhi Jois, taught a precise method of asana and pranayama practice that accesses the supreme state of liberated existence, which is mentioned on the Yoga Sutras. He named this style of yoga practice Ashtanga Yoga.

This method of asana practice was described in the Yoga Korunta, a sacred text composed by Vamana Rishi. The Yoga Korunta has been passed down in the tradition of Guru Shishya Parampara—a succession of teachers and disciples—by Guru Rama Mohan Brahmachari to Sri T Krishnamacharya, who entrusted it to his disciple Sri K Pattabhi Jois in 1927. The Yoga Korunta emphasizes a precise method of asana practice, which includes hundreds of asanas and a specific pranayama sequence. In the text, it is instructed that vinyasa is an essential element of asana practice.

Vinyasa intimately links the inhaling and exhaling breath to the movement of the body in and out of the postures. The vinyasa or continuous movement between the postures creates an internal heat that eases the body into the various asanas. In the Yoga Korunta it is specifically advised not to practice asana without vinyasa.

The Ashtanga Yoga practice includes hundreds of asanas, which are divided into primary, intermediate and advanced series.

The primary series or Yoga Chikitsa, is designed to eliminate disease. The intermediate series, which is referred to as Nadi Shodhana, purifies the nadies or subtle energy channels underlying the physical form. The advanced series or Sthira Bhaga, consists of 3 or 4 series of advanced asanas, that stabilize inner radiance. Sthira means steady and Bhaga is an ancient God of love and prosperity.

In Ashtanga Yoga, the asanas are practiced in sequential order, and are preceded and concluded by a vinyasa. Each practice, of any series, begins with Surya Namaskara, a sequence of asanas also known as Sun Salutations. There are two types of Surya Namaskara—A and B—that are repeated five times each prior to practicing individual asanas. Surya Namaskara is essentially a series of vinyasas; since each asana, except for Adho Mukha Shvanasana, downward facing dog posture, is held for only a moment at the end of either the inhaling or exhaling breath, while the alternating inhaling and exhaling breath is stretched throughout the movements between one asana and the next. Adho Mukha Shvanasana is the only asana, which is held for five breaths in each Surya Namaskara.

The standing asanas are the first set of asanas following Surya Namaskaras A and B. Each standing asana is held for five to eight breaths. A specific set of vinyasas guide the body in and out of each standing asana, back to Samastitihi, a precise standing pose with the feet together and hands at the side known also as equal standing. After practicing the standing asanas, the asanas that are specific to either the primary, intermediate or advanced series are practiced. These asanas are each linked by a specific vinyasa, that most commonly, consists of one segment of the Surya Namaskara, that includes the three Asanas, Chaturanga Dandasana(four limbed staff asana), Urdhva Mukha Shvanasana(upward facing dog posture) and Adho Mukha Shvanasana(downward facing dog posture). The finishing

INTRODUCTION

sequence is practiced after completing the asanas unique to either the primary, intermediate or advanced series. The finishing asanas are 15 in total and include Urdhva Dhanurasana (upward facing bow posture), Sarvangasana (shoulder stand), Shirshasana (headstand) and Padmasana (lotus posture). These asanas are linked by another unique set of vinyasas.

As described, the body remains within either an asana or a vinyasa throughout the entire length of the Ashtanga Yoga practice, consisting of between 60 and 70 asanas each day. The vinyasa element of the practice creates cardiovascular fitness, maintains warmth in the body and joints, and induces a continuous meditative awareness.

When starting this practice, one begins with the Surya Namaskara. Then, the standing asanas, the primary series asanas and the finishing asanas are introduced. The order of the asanas is such that each one prepares the practitioner by opening the body to the next. After several years of consistent practice of the primary series, the postures of the intermediate series are added one at a time—to the primary series, prior to the finishing asanas. When two thirds of the asanas of the intermediate series are added to the primary series, the primary series is dropped and practiced only once a week. The other days of the week, two thirds of the intermediate series is practiced and the remaining third of the asanas are added one at a time. After several years of practice of the intermediate series, the advanced series asanas are added one at a time to the intermediate series, in the same manner as the intermediate series asanas were added to the primary series.

In this way hundreds of asanas are integrated into the body of the practitioner over numerous decades of practice. This practice is to be continued throughout a lifetime. The Ashtanga Yoga practice purifies and strengthens the body, mind and sense organs, which ensures a healthy, long life to its practitioner.

Within the practice, the asana and vinyasa are deepened and refined by Trishtana. Trishtana is the threefold placement of awareness during asana practice. Trishtana includes awareness of asana (the posture), pranayama (the breath), and drishti (the looking place).

Asana is translated as "seat" or "posture." The original meaning of the word asana is derived from the stool a yoga practitioner sat on while meditating. In common usage, asana refers to posture. Asana practice draws consciousness into the body, as the practitioner directs the body into the asanas. Awareness is to be directed into the asanas, throughout the practice.

Pranayama is translated from Sanskrit as "breath control." A specific breathing technique, called Ujjayi (pronounced "oo-ja-yee") Pranayama is practiced throughout the asanas and vinyasas. Ujjayi Pranayama is a deep, rhythmic breathing technique that is characterized by a slight contraction in the throat. This slight contraction creates a subtle sound, similar to the sound of the ocean, throughout the length of the inhale and exhale. Ujjayi Pranayama increases the lung capacity, oxygenates the blood and stills the mind. The contraction in the throat slows down the breath, by reducing the volume of air that passes in and out of the lungs throughout any given length of time. During asana practice, the length of the inhale should equal the length of the exhale and the breath should never be held. When practicing Ujjayi Pranayama, a continuous, smooth, subtle sound is produced throughout the cycle of the breath. By listening to the sound of the breath and keeping awareness of the breath, the mind becomes clear.

The third aspect of Trishtana is drishti. Drishti is the looking place designated to each asana and vinyasa. There are a total of nine drishtis: nasa (nose), urdhva (upward), ajna (third eye), pada (foot), hasta (hand), angusta (thumb), nabi (Navel) and two parshva (to the left and to the right). Practicing drishti, places the head and aligns the spine correctly in the asana and throughout the vinyasa. Drishti

INTRODUCTION

eliminates distractions and increases the ability of the mind to concentrate.

Trishtana, the three-fold placement of awareness, increases the potency of asana practice.

In addition to Ujjayi Pranayama and drishti, the Ashtanga method of asana practice is accompanied by control and awareness of the bandhas. Bandha translates from Sanskrit as "lock" or "seal." There are three bandhas, each of which involves muscular contraction. Mula Bandha, the root lock, is activated by a contraction of the pelvic floor. Uddiyana Bandha, the flying lock, is activated by drawing the portion above and below the navel back to the spine. Jalandhara Bandha, the net lock, is practiced by contracting the throat and drawing the chin firmly against the sternum.

The three bandhas direct the movement of subtle energy in the body. In the Hatha Yoga Pradipika, a classic Sanskrit manual on yoga, it is mentioned that Mula Bandha moves Apana Vayu (the downward moving breath) upward into the fire region of the navel. This intensifies the heat, which arouses Kundalini. Kundalini is the dormant energy that lies coiled at the base of the spine. Uddiyana Bandha moves prana—vital energy—into the Sushumna Nadi, or central channel, extending along the length of the spine. Jalandhara Bandha keeps the Amrita—the nectar of immortality situated in the brain—from dripping down and being consumed by the fire in the navel region. The contraction in the throat closes the Ida and Pingala Nadis—the solar and lunar energy channels, which originate in the two nostrils—and moves prana into the Sushumna Nadi. When prana moves freely in the Sushumna Nadi, then the fire in the navel region and Kundalini can be taken there. When the awakened Kundalini moves into the Sushumna Nadi, ultimate liberation is revealed to the yoga practitioner.

Mula Bandha is engaged throughout the asana practice. Uddiyana and Jalandhara Bandha are practiced during pranayama practice and occasionally during asana practice. The bandhas are cultivated over many years of practice. They deepen the asanas and conserve the energy of the yoga practitioner.

The application of vinyasa, Ujjayi Pranayama, drishti and bandhas to asana practice is what makes the Ashtanga method safe and highly effective. These principles are applied throughout the primary, intermediate and advanced series of postures.

Ashtanga Vinyasa Yoga is to be learned under the guidance of an experienced practitioner and qualified teacher. Even though it seems that the Ashtanga method prescribes the same practice to everyone, the practice is individualized when a qualified teacher oversees when new postures are added and the length of time each practitioner is advised to practice a series of postures. This individualization accounts for the need to strengthen unique weaknesses in each practitioner.

The practice is to take place six days a week. Saturdays are the traditional rest days. The other days on which practice is suspended are the new and full moon days and for women the first three days of menstruation. The practice is also progressively reduced during pregnancy and then suspended for up to three months after giving birth.

It is instructed by Patanjali in the Yoga Sutras that in order for yoga practice to be firmly grounded, it must be cultivated correctly over an extended, uninterrupted period of time. In this case, in order to be able to access the asanas of the primary, intermediate and advanced series, it is necessary to practice on a regular basis for ten to fifteen consecutive years, again, under the guidance of an experienced instructor.

Practicing Ashtanga Vinyasa Yoga five or six days a week for 10 to 15 consecutive years, under the guidance of an experienced instructor, not only enables one access to the asanas of all three series mentioned, but it also encourages an experience of pure consciousness, the elimination of disease and a content emotional state.

OM

Vande Gurunam Charanaravinde

Sandarashita Svatma Sukhavabodhe

Nishreyase Jangalikayamane

Samsara Halahala Mohashantyai

Abahu Purusakaram

Sankhacakrasi Dharinam

Sahasra Sirasam Svetam

Pranamami Patanjalim

OM

INVOCATION

Om is the syllable representing Ishvara. Ishvara is a special being who is untouched by afflictions, actions or the results of action and is thus considered the seed of all knowing. Ishvara is the first and foremost Guru who is unconditioned by time. Om is to be chanted, while the mind rests on its full significance. When chanted in this manner, it removes obstacles to the knowledge of the true self.

Translation:
I worship the lotus feet of the linage of gurus
Thereby awakening the happiness of the self revealed
Acting like the jungle physician
To pacify the poison from the delusion of conditioned existence
(Source: Yoga Taravalli by Adi Shankaracharya)

Translation:
I invoke the sage Patanjali,
Who has a thousand radiant white heads.
He assumes the form of a man until the arms,
Which hold a conch shell, a chakra (or wheel) and a sword.
(Source: Traditional Chant)

Surya Namaskara is the ultimate
worship of the Sun God

Sri K Pattabhi Jois

SURYA NAMASKARA

Asana practice is commenced with Surya Namaskara. Traditionally Surya Namaskara is practiced facing the rising sun. This is the ideal time for asana practice, early in the morning before breakfast. If one does practice later in the day, it is best to wait 2 to 3 hours after a meal to practice asanas. Surya Namaskara consists primarily of vinyasa, the only asana which is held for five breaths is Adho Mukha Shvanasana, downward facing dog. The practice of Surya Namaskara creates heat in the body, awakens the breathing system and offers a wide range of movement to the body. In the Ashtanga Vinyasa System, there are two types of Surya Namaskara—A and B—each of which is practiced five times. Surya Namaskara A is composed of five asanas, to which two asanas are added in Surya Namaskara B.

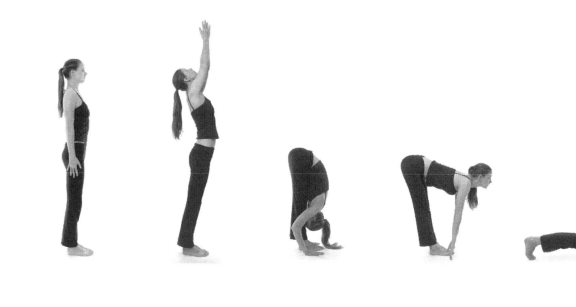

SAMASTITIHI   EKAM   DVE   TRINI   CHATVARI

SURYA NAMASKARA A

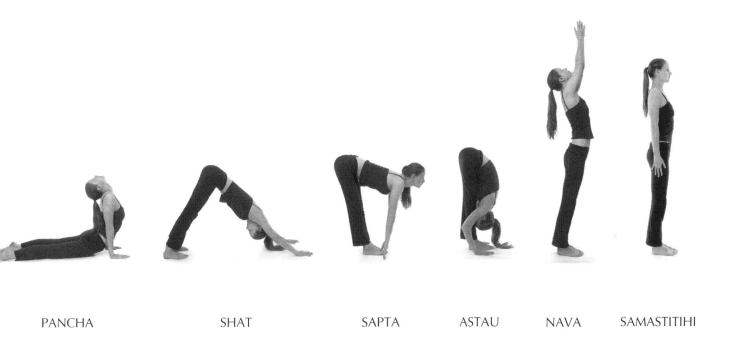

PANCHA   SHAT   SAPTA   ASTAU   NAVA   SAMASTITIHI

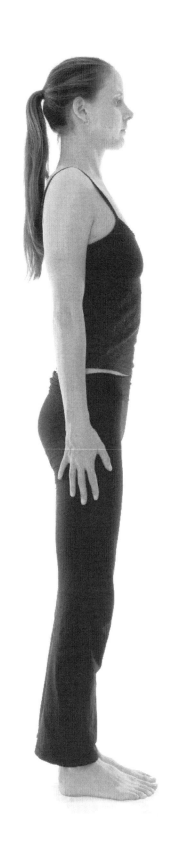

ASHTANGA YOGA

SAMASTITIHI

The first asana of Surya Namaskara A is Samastitihi (equal standing). To enter Samastitihi, place the feet together so that the insides of the feet touch, straighten the legs and spine, keep the head level, draw the shoulders back and allow the arms to extend down either side of the body. Soften the eyes and gaze towards the tip of the nose—nasa drishti.

Engage Mula Bandha, by contracting the muscles in the pelvic floor. Continue to hold this contraction throughout the asana practice. Then, begin Oujaii Pranayama by slightly contracting the throat to create a soft sound on the inhaling and exhaling breath. Slow down; deepen and lengthen the breath. The length of the inhale should equal the length of the exhale. Lift the sternum slightly on the inhale and draw the navel back to the spine on the exhale.

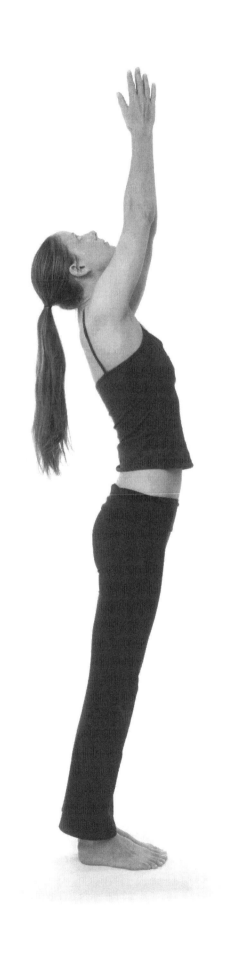

EKAM

Enter the first (ekam) asana on the inhaling breath. Keep
the arms straight and rotate them externally , as you raise
the hands up over the head until the palms touch. Lift the
sternum slightly and tilt the head back in order to look at
the thumbs—angusta drishti.

Uttanasana

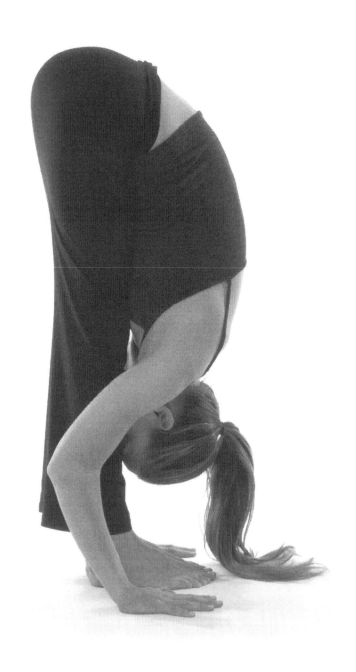

DVE

The second (dve) asana is Uttanasana, a standing forward bend. On the exhaling breath, lower the arms out to the sides and down, placing the palms of the hands on the floor on either sides of the feet, draw the hips back slightly and fold the torso forward and down, until the chest touches the legs. Keep the legs straight and draw the head in towards the legs and look towards the nose—nasa drishti.

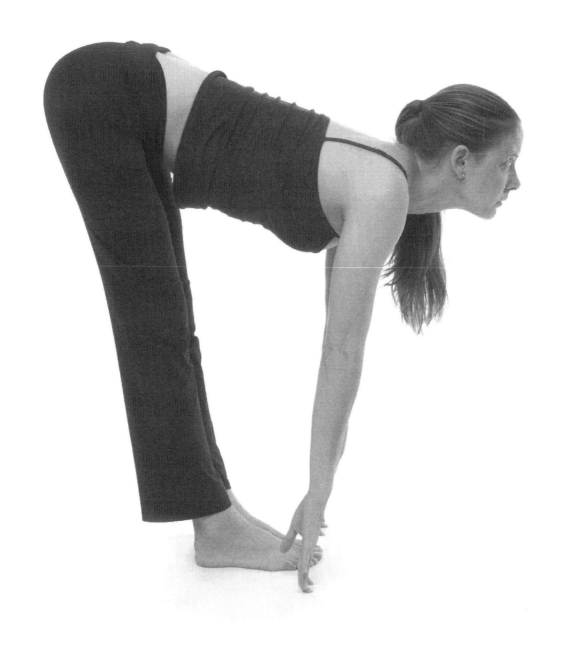

TRINI

Enter the third (trini) asana on the inhaling breath. Lift the head until the spine and arms straighten. Keep the finger-tips in contact with the floor on either side of the feet. Lift the sit bones and re-straighten the legs. Direct the gaze up into the forehead—anja drishti.

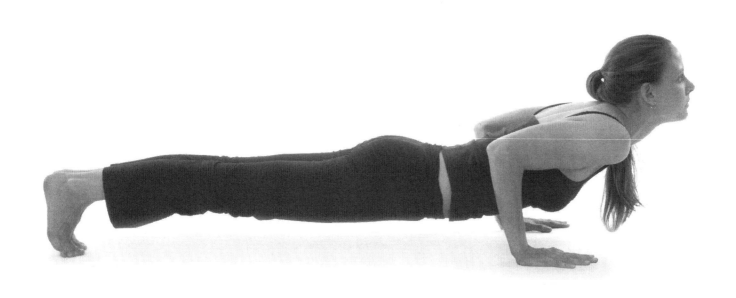

CHATVARI

The fourth (chatvari) asana is Chaturanga Dandasana, the four limbed staff posture. Enter this position by pressing the palms of the hands into the floor on either side of the feet. Keep the head lifted and hop back on the exhaling breath, by lifting the hips slightly and keeping the legs straight as the feet extend back. As you hop back, bend the elbows, pulling them in toward the torso, and flex the feet in order to land on the toes. Keeping the head lifted, stretch the chin forward and gaze towards the tip of the nose—nasa drishti.

Urdhva Mukha Shvanasana

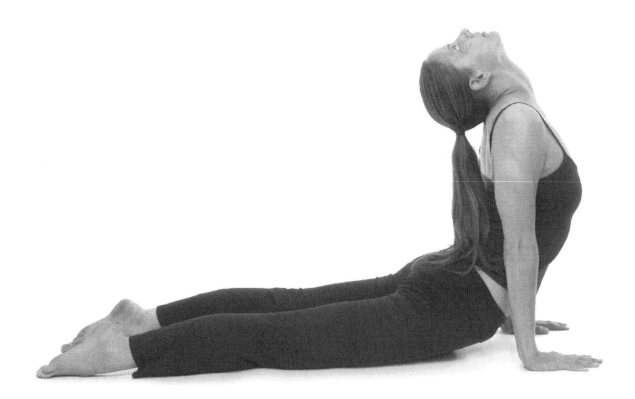

PANCHA

The fifth (pancha) asana is Urdhva Mukha Shvanasana, upward facing dog posture. Inhale, pull the ribcage forward and up and straighten the arms. Roll forward over the toes until they point straight back. Keep the arms and legs straight and arch the spine back by pressing the tops of the feet into the floor—the body's weight is on the palms and the tops of the feet only. Tilt the head back, and look up into the forehead—ajna drishti).

Adho Mukha Shvanasana

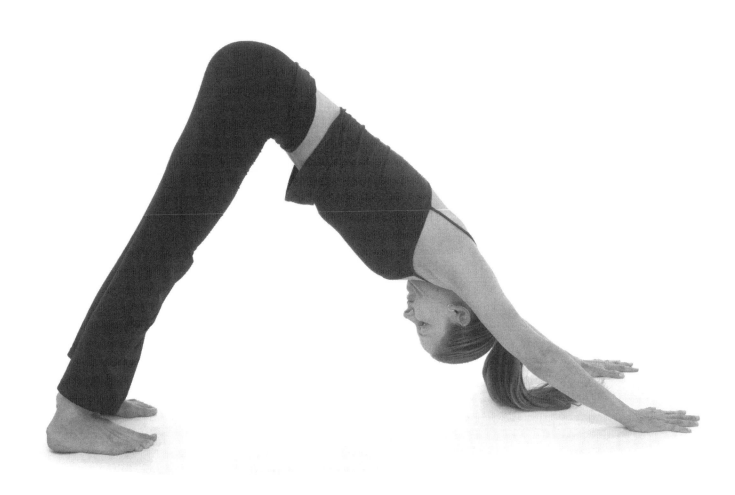

SHAT

The sixth (shat) asana is Adho Mukha Shvanasana (downward facing dog posture). Move into this asana on the exhaling breath. Keeping the arms straight, press the palms of the hands down and away into the floor. Lift the hips, reach the heels back, roll over the toes and press the heels down into the floor. Pull the spine back with the hips and create a straight line with the torso and arms from the hands to the hips. The palms of the hands should be shoulder width apart and the feet hip width apart with the toes pointing forward. Drop the head through the arms, draw the chin in towards the chest, and shift the gaze towards the navel—nabi drishti. Hold this asana for five smooth, deep breaths.

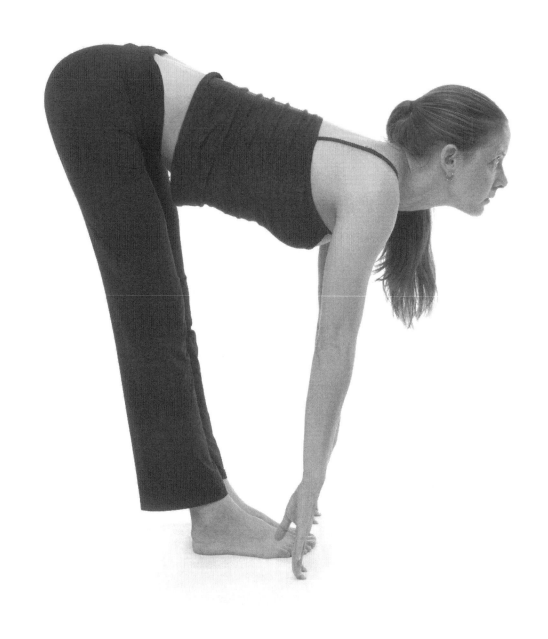

SAPTA

Enter the seventh (sapta) asana at the end of the fifth exhale. Bend the knees slightly, hop the feet forward between the hands and straighten the legs by lifting the hips. In the air, bring the feet together, so that the insides of the feet touch, when the soles of the feet land on the floor. Inhale, straighten the legs, spine and arms, keeping the fingertips in contact with the floor. Lift the head and return the gaze to the center of the forehead—ajna drishti.

Uttanasana

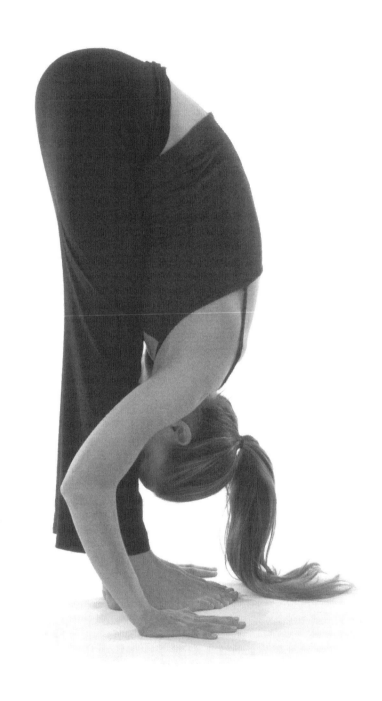

ASHTAU

The eighth (ashtau) asana is Uttanasana (standing forward bend). On the exhale, keeping the legs straight, fold the torso down to the legs, draw the head in towards the legs and look towards the nose—nasa drishti.

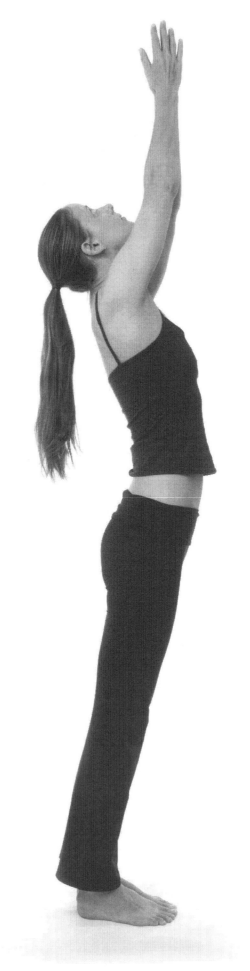

NAVA

To enter the ninth (nava) asana, lift the head, inhale and
raise the torso back up to standing with a straight spine as
you reach the arms out and up over the head until the palms
of the hands touch. Tilt the head back and shift the gaze to
the thumbs—angusta drishti.

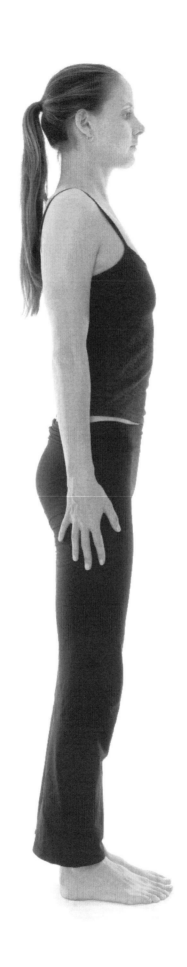

SAMASTITIHI

The tenth (dasha) asana is Samastitihi (equal standing). On the exhale, extend the arms out and down to either side of the torso, drop the chin until it is parallel to the floor and shift the gaze to the tip of the nose—nasa drishti.

Repeat Surya Namaskara A five times. After exhaling into Samastitihi at the end of the fifth Surya Namaskara A enter the first asana of Surya Namaskara B as follows.

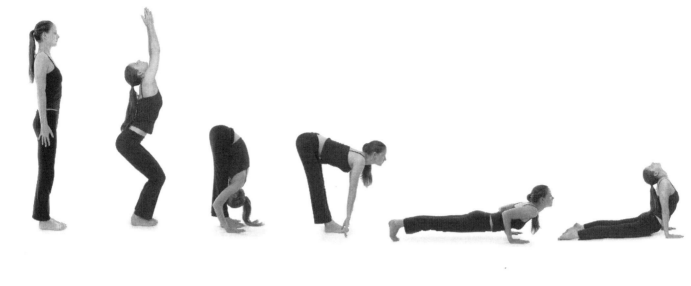

SAMASTITIHI   EKAM   DVE   TRINI   CHATVARI   PANCHA

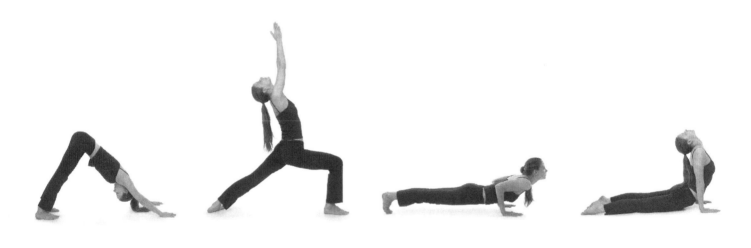

SHAT   SAPTA   ASHTAU   NAVA

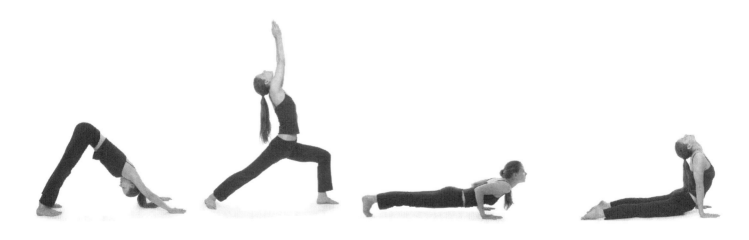

DASHA   EKADASHA   DVADASHA   TRAYODASHA

ASHTANGA YOGA

SURYA NAMASKARA B

Surya Namaskara B includes two additional Asanas, Utkatasana (the
fierce posture) and Virabhadrasana (the warrior posture).

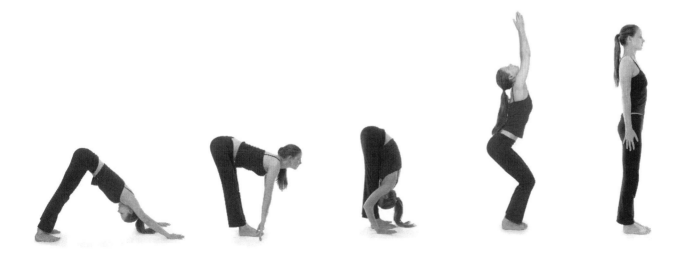

CHATURDASHA   PANCHADASHA   SODASHA   SAPTADASHA   SAMASTITIHI

Utkatasana

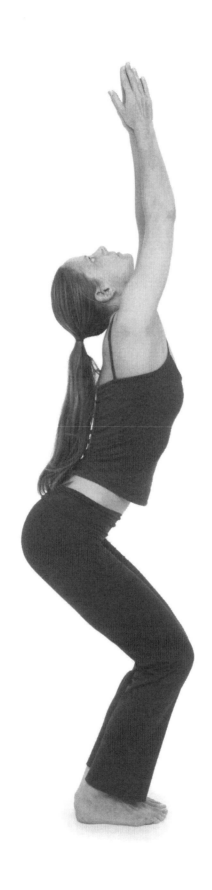

EKAM

The first (ekam) position of Surya Namaskara B is
Utkatasana (the fierce posture). To enter Utkatasana, bend
the knees deeply. Inhale, raise the arms, keeping them
straight, and join the palms of the hands above the head, so
that the arms are perpendicular to the floor. Tilt the head
back and look up to the thumbs—angusta drishti. Keep the
insides of the feet in contact with each other and press the
knees together gently.

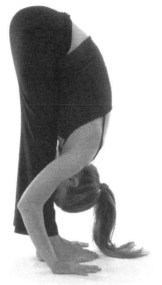

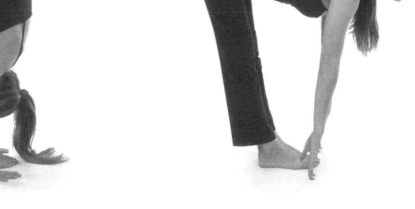

DVE   TRINI

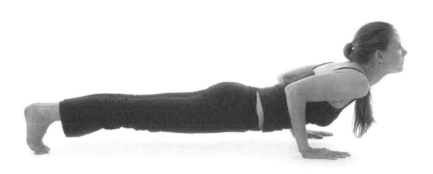

CHATVARI

The second (dve) asana is Uttanasana. Exhale, straighten the legs, reach the arms out and down, fold the torso forward and down, and place the palms of the hands on the floor on either side of the feet. Draw the head in towards the legs and look towards the nose—nasa drishti.

Then, inhale, lift the head until the arms and spine straighten keeping the fingers in contact with the floor, and focus the gaze to the forehead—ajna drishti.

Exhale, hop back and lower the body down into Chaturanga Dandasana. Inhale, lift the ribcage forward and up, tilt the head back, press the tops of the feet into the floor and arch the spine into Urdhva Mukha Shvanasana. Exhale lift the hips back and up into Adho Mukha Shvanasana.

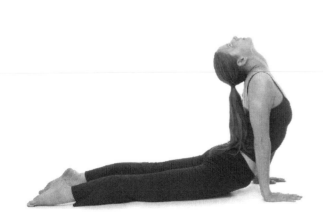

PANCHA

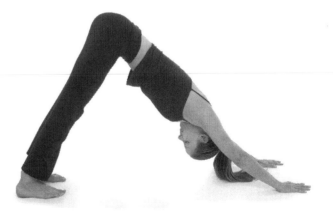

SHAT

Virabhadrasana

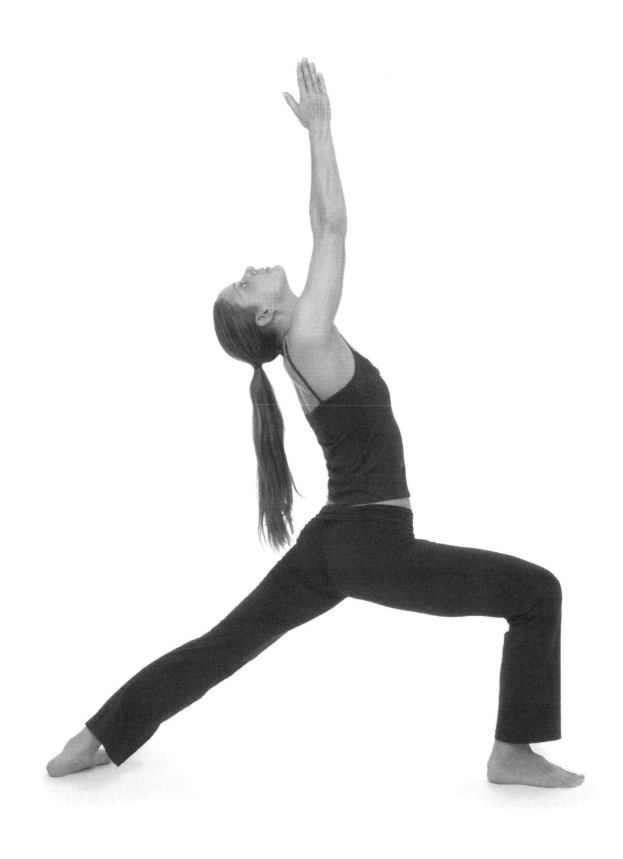

SAPTA

Virabhadrasana (the warrior posture) on the right side, is the seventh (sapta) asana of Surya Namaskara B.

From Adho Mukha Shvanasana, keeping the left leg straight, rotate the left leg externally, press the left heel into the floor and step the right foot forward between the hands. Drop the hips, and bend the right leg until the knee extends slightly forward over the ankle. Extend back into the outside of the left foot, keeping the left leg straight. Inhale, lift the torso, straighten the arms and reach them out and up over the head until the palms of the hands join above the head. Lift the sternum, tilt the head back and rest the gaze on the thumbs—angusta drishti.

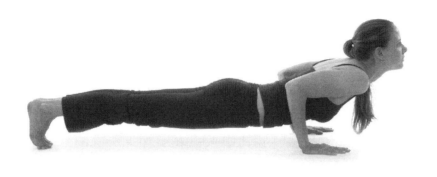

ASHTAU

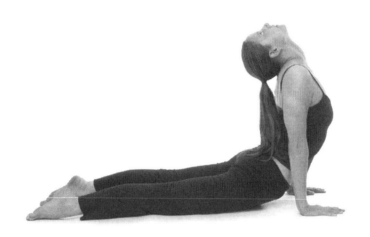

NAVA

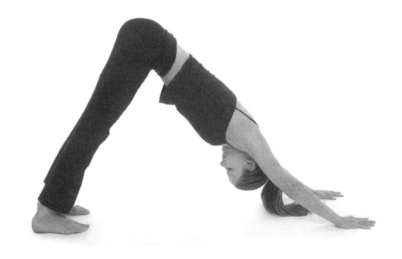

DASHA

From Virabhadrasana on the right side, exhale, fold the torso forward and place the palms of the hands on the floor on either side of the right foot. Rotate the left leg internally and lift the left heel, keeping the left leg straight. Step the right leg back next to the left leg and lower the body down into Chaturanga Dandasana. Inhale into Urdhva Mukha Shvanasana. Exhale into Adho Mukha Shvanasana.

Virabhadrasana

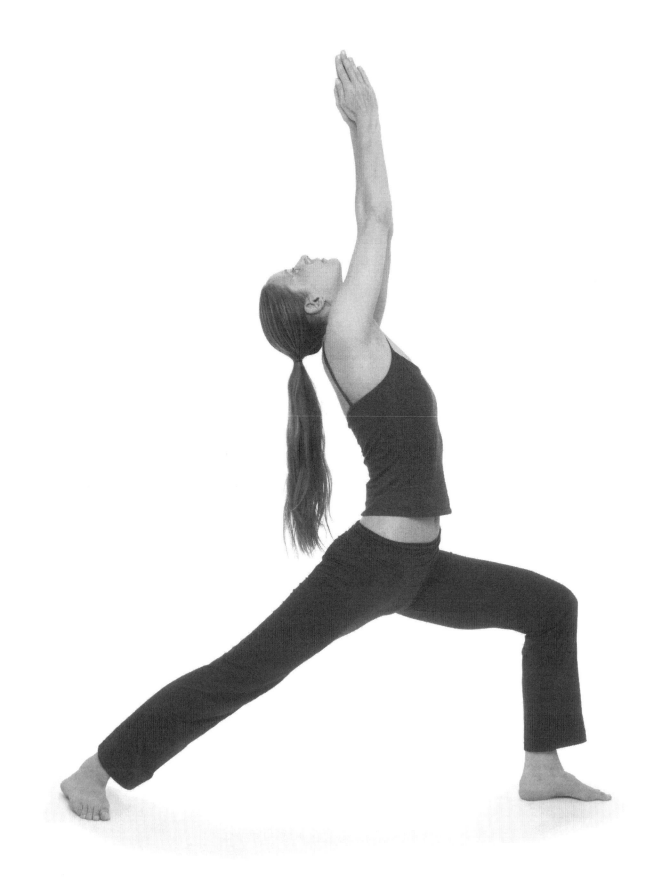

EKADASHA

Virabhadrasana (the warrior posture), on the left side is the eleventh (ekadasa) asana of Surya Namaskara B.

From Adho Mukha Shvanasana, keeping the right leg straight, rotate the right leg externally and press the right heel into the floor. Step the left foot forward between the hands. Lower the hips and bend the left leg until the left knee extends forward over the left ankle. Extend back into the right leg and press the outside of the right foot into the floor. Inhaling, raise the torso, straighten the arms, reach them out and up to join the palms of the hands above the head. Lift the sternum, tilt the head back and look up to the thumbs (Angusta Drishti).

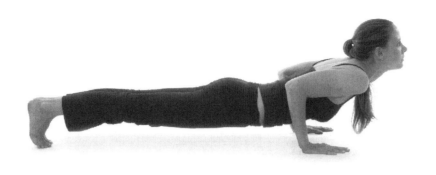

DVADASHA

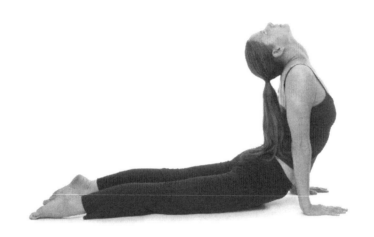

TRAYODASHA

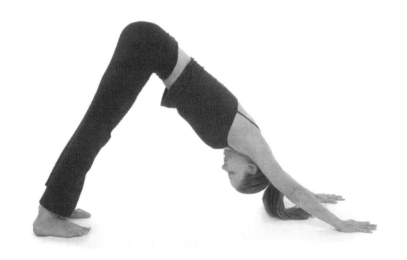

CHATURDASHA

ASHTANGA YOGA

From Virabhadrasana on the left side, exhale, fold the torso forward and place the palms of the hands on the floor on either side of the left foot. Keeping the right leg straight, rotate the right leg internally and lift the heel. Step the left foot back next to the right foot and lower the body down into Chaturanga Dandasana. Inhale lift the rib cage forward and up into Urdhva Mukha Shvanasana. Exhale, lift the hips and pull the spine back and up into Adho Mukha Shvanasana. Draw the chin into the chest and shift the gaze towards the navel (Nabi Drishti). Hold this last Adho Mukha Shvanasana in Surya Namaskara B for five deep, long breaths.

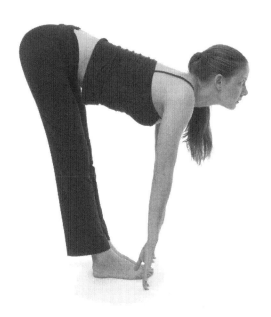

PANCHADASHA

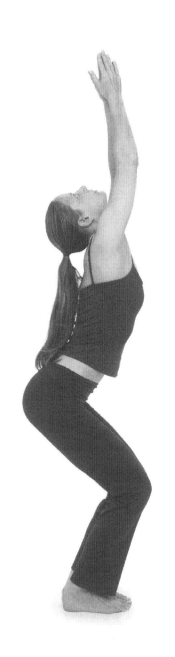

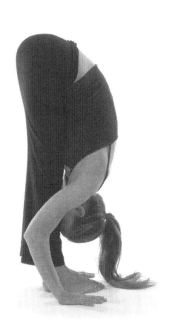

SHODASHA

SAPTADASHA

At the end of the fifth exhale, bend the knees slightly and
hop forward, lifting the hips and keeping the legs straight.
In the air, bring the feet together, so that the insides of
the feet touch when the soles of the feet land on the floor.
Inhale, lift the head and straighten the legs, spine and arms.
Keep the fingertips in contact with the floor, and return the
gaze to the center of the forehead—ajna drishti..

Exhale, and fold the torso forward and down into
Uttanasana.

Then enter Utkatasana, by bending the knees deeply
and press them together gently. Inhale, raise the torso,
straighten the arms and reach the hands out and up over the
head until the palms join. Tilt the head back, and look up
to the thumbs—angusta drishti.

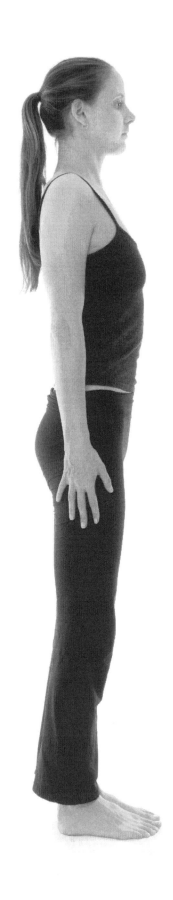

SAMASTITIHI

Exhale, straighten the legs, reach the arms out and lower
them down to either side of the torso and lower the chin
into Samastitihi. Look towards the tip of the nose—nasa
drishti.

Repeat Surya Namaskara B five times. Surya Namaskara B
is more challenging than Surya Namaskara A. At first you
may need to take an extra breath when stepping into Virabhadrasana, but once you are familiarized with the postures
and Vinyasa of Surya Namaskara B, avoid taking extra
breaths.

The practice of Surya Namaskara A and B creates internal
heat, awakens the breathing system and induces a calm
meditative state in preparation for the remainder of the
practice.

STANDING ASANAS

The standing asanas are practiced after completing Surya Namaskara A and B. The Surya Namaskaras and the standing asanas are practiced prior to the asanas that are unique to the Primary, Intermediate or Advanced Series. The standing asanas prepare the body for the subsequent asanas by directing prana (the subtle energy underlying the physical form) down the legs and connect the body to the Earth.

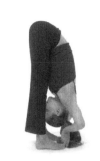

PADANGUSTASANA

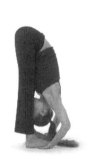

PADA HASTASANA

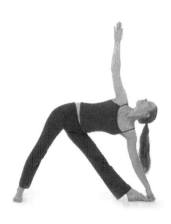

UTTHITA TRIKONASANA

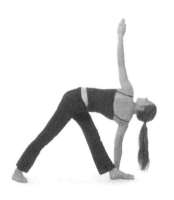

PARIVRTTA TRIKONASANA

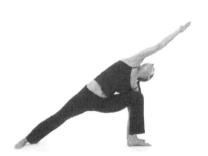

UTTHITA PARSHVAKONASANA

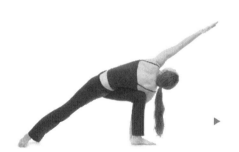

PARIVRTTA PARSHVAKONASANA

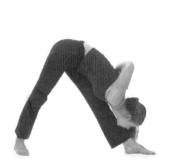

PARSHVOTTANSANA

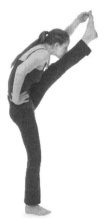

A

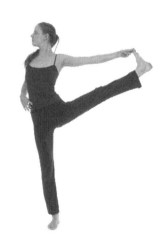

B

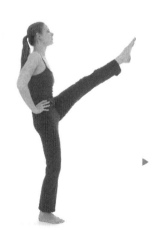

C

UTTHITA HASTA PADANGUSTASANA

STANDING ASANAS

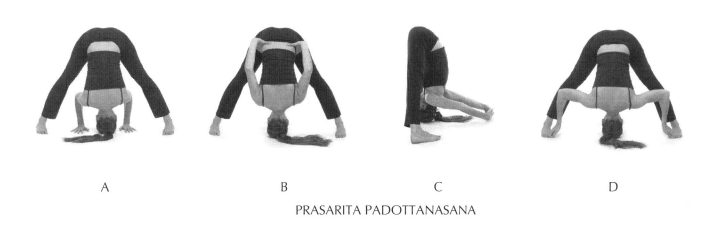

A   B   C   D

PRASARITA PADOTTANASANA

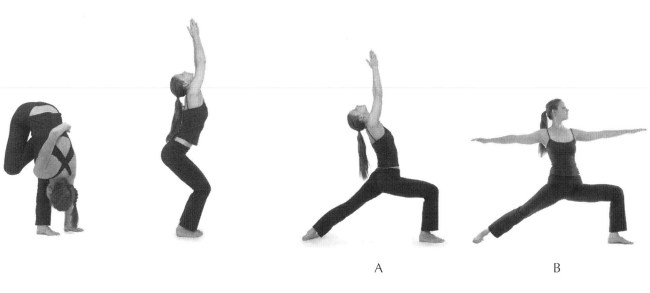

ARDHA BADDHA   UTKATASANA   VIRABHADRASANA
PADMOTTANASANA

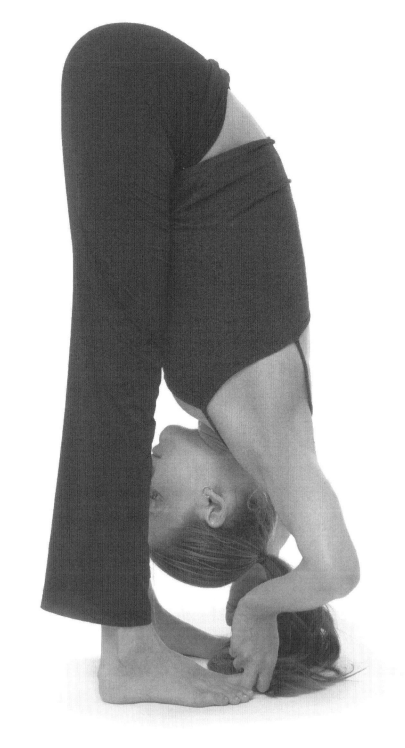

ASHTANGA YOGA

PADANGUSTHASANA

Hop the feet hip width apart and place the hands on the hips. Inhale, lift the chest. Exhale, fold the torso forward and down to the legs, keeping the legs straight. Lower the arms and encircle the big toes with the first two fingers, completing the circle with the thumbs. Inhale lift the head, until the arms and torso straighten. Exhale, touch the torso to the legs using the arms and engaging the abdominal muscles. Drop the head and pull it in between the legs. Look toward the tip of the nose—nasa drishti. Remain here for five long, deep breaths.

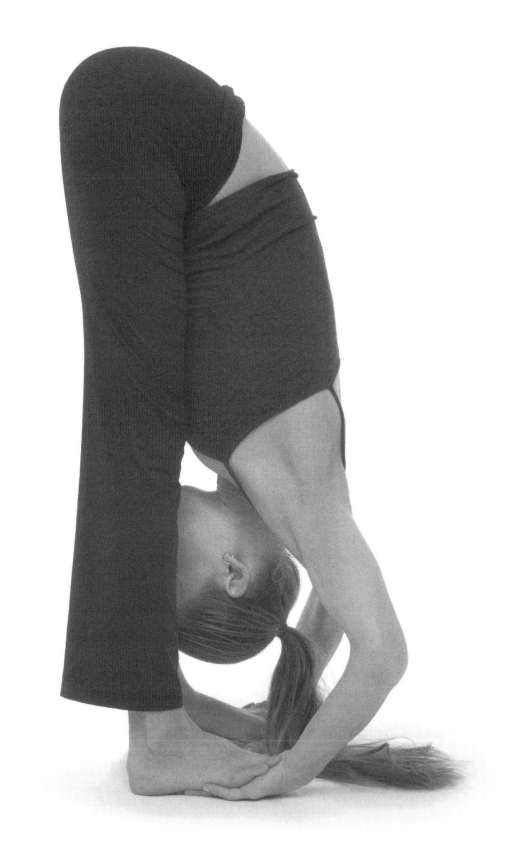

PADA HASTASANA

Inhale lift the head until the arms and torso straighten. Release the grip around the big toes and slide the hands underneath the feet, with the palms of the hands facing up. Exhale, draw the torso back down until it touches the legs using the arms and abdominal muscles. Drop the head and pull it between the legs, looking toward the tip of the nose—nasa drishti. Stay here for five deep breaths.

Then inhale and lift the head until the arms and torso straighten. Exhale, place the hands on the hips. Inhale, raise the torso up to standing, keeping a straight spine. Exhale, hop the feet back together into Samastitihi and bring the palms of the hands together into Anjali Mudra in front of the chest.

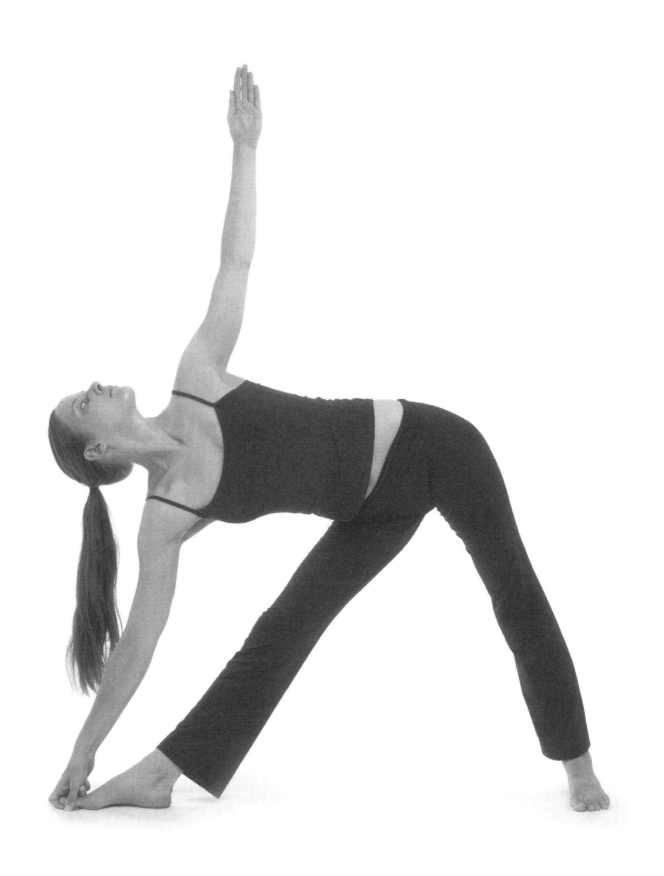

UTTHITA TRIKONASANA

Enter Utthita Trikonasana by jumping the feet three to four feet apart, 90 degrees to the right and stretch the arms out to the sides on the inhaling breath. Then rotate the right foot and leg 90 degrees to the right so that it is perpendicular to the left foot. Exhale, tilt the torso to the right over the right leg, by tilting the hips and reach down toward the right foot with the right hand, keeping the arms straight. Encircle the right big toe with the first two fingers of the right hand, completing the circle with the thumb. Reach the left hand up toward the ceiling. Rotate the head to the left and look toward the left thumb—angusta drishti. Stay here for five deep, even breaths.

Inhale, reach the left arm up and to the left as you raise the torso back up to standing and lift the right arm out to the right. Repeat the position on the other side—rotate the right foot 90 degrees to the left and the left foot forward 90 degrees to the left. Exhale, tilt the torso to the left over the left leg, by tilting the hips and reach toward the left foot with the left hand, keeping the arms straight. Encircle the left big toe with the first two fingers of the left hand, completing the circle with the thumb. Reach the right arm up to the ceiling. Rotate the head to the right and rest the gaze on the right thumb—angusta drishti. Hold Uttitha Trikonasana on the left side for five deep breaths. After completing the fifth exhale, inhale and stretch the right arm up and to the right, raising the torso back to standing and extending the left arm out to the left.

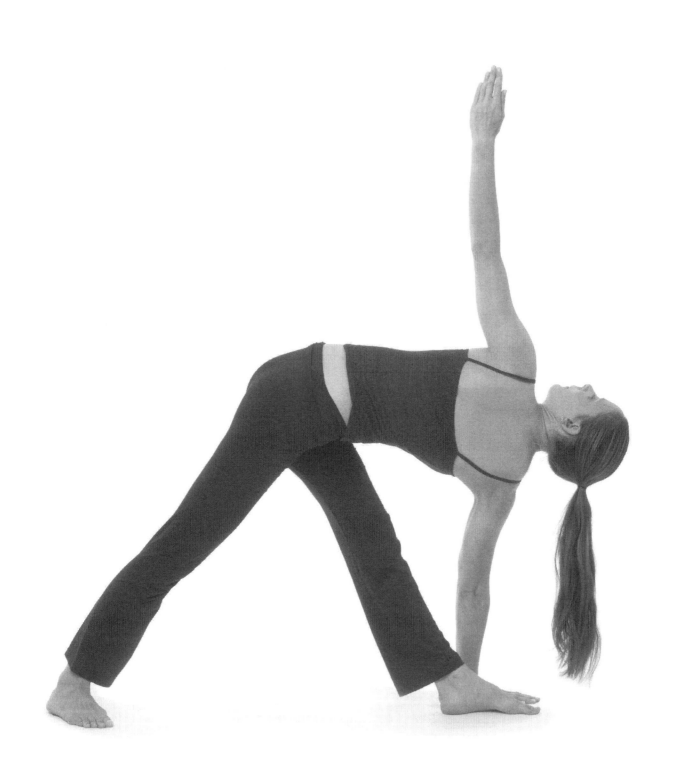

PARIVRTTA TRIKONASANA

Starting in Samastitihi jump the feet three to four feet apart 90 degrees to the right, extend the left arm up to the ceiling and drop the right arm down to the side of the torso, keeping the arms straight. Rotate the left leg and foot 45 degrees to the right and the right foot and right leg 90 degrees to the right. Exhale, lowering the torso down over the right leg until it is parallel to the floor. Reach the left arm, keeping the arm straight, forward and down, placing the left hand firmly on the floor to the right of the right foot as you reach the right arm straight, back and up to the ceiling. Inhale and twist the torso to the right by pressing the palm of the left hand into the floor. Rotate the head to the right and rest the gaze on the right thumb—angusta drishti.

Stay in Parivrtta Trikonasana on the right side for five deep breaths.

Inhale, as you raise the torso back up to standing and reach the left arm forward, up over the head and down to the left side and the right arm back, down and then forward and up. Rotate the hips, legs and feet to the left. Pull the left hip back, rotating the left foot straight ahead to the left and the right foot 45 degrees to the right. Exhale, lowering the torso down over the left leg until it is parallel to the floor and reaching the right arm straight, forward and down to place the palm of the right hand on the floor to the left of the left foot as you reach the left arm straight, back and up to the ceiling. Inhale, and twist the torso to the left, by pressing the palm of the right hand into the floor. Rotate the head to the left, and rest the gaze on the left thumb— angusta drishti.

Stay in Parivrtta Trikonasana on the left side for five deep breaths.

Then, inhale, reach the right arm forward, up and out to the right as you lift the torso back up to standing. Rotate the hips to the right as you reach the left arm back down and out to the left. Exhale, hop the feet back together, ninety degrees to the left into Samastitihi as you place the palms of the hands together in front of the chest in Anjali Mudra.

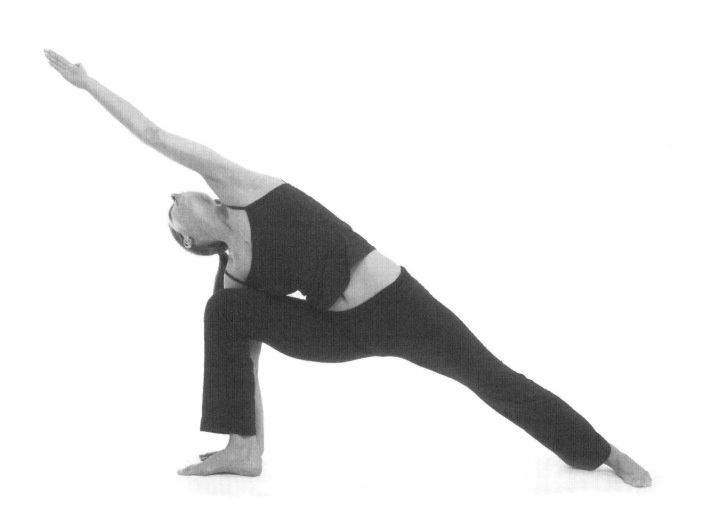

UTTHITA PARSHVAKONASANA

Inhale, jump the feet four to five feet apart 90 degrees to the right and extend the arms out to the sides at shoulder height. Turn the right foot 90 degrees to the right and extend the left heel slightly out to the left. Exhale, bend the right knee until the knee extends out over the ankle. Place the palm of the right hand on the floor to the right of the right foot and reach the left arm, keeping it straight, forward and up over the head away from the left foot with the palm of the left hand facing down. Create a straight line with the body, from the outside of the left foot to the left fingertips, by adjusting the width of the feet. Tilt the head back and look at the palm of the left hand—hasta drishti. Stay here for five breaths.

Inhale, reach the left arm up to the ceiling and down to the left as you raise the torso back up to standing and the right arm out to the right. Straighten the right leg, turning the right foot forward 90 degrees to the left and the left foot 90 degrees to the left. Exhale, bend the left leg until the knee extends out over the ankle. Place the palm of the left hand on the floor to the left of the left foot and reach the right arm, keeping it straight, forward and up over the head, away from the right foot with the palm of the right hand facing down. Create a straight line with the body, from the outside of the right foot to the right fingertips, by adjusting the width of the feet. Tilt the head back and look at the palm of the right hand—hasta drishti. Stay here for five breaths.

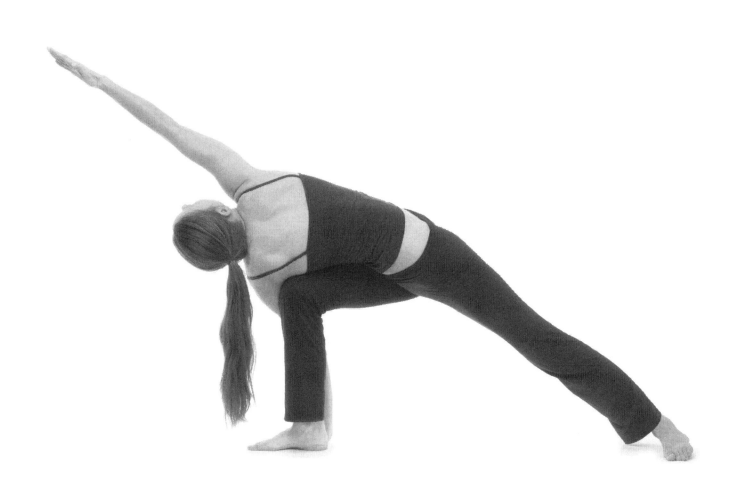

PARIVRTTA PARSHVAKONASANA

Inhale, reach the right arm up to the ceiling and out to the right as you raise the torso back up to standing and lift the left arm straight out to the left. Straighten the left leg, turn the left foot forward, 90 degrees to the right and the right foot 90 degrees to the right. Rotate the hips to the right, raise the left arm up to the ceiling and lower the right arm down to the side of the torso. Exhale, bend the right leg until the right knee extends over the ankle, extend the left heel back behind the left toes, reaching the left arm forward and down to the right of the right knee. Place the palm of the left hand on the floor to the right of the right foot. Twist the torso to the left and reach the right arm, keeping it straight, forward and up over the head away from the left foot, with the palm of the hand facing down. Create a straight line with the body from the outside of the left foot to the right finger tips. Tilt the head back and look at the palm of the right hand--hasta drishti. Remain in Parivrtta Parshvakonasana on the right side for five deep breaths.

Inhale, raise the torso back up to standing and straighten the right leg, as you reach the left arm forward, up and out to the left and extend the right arm out to the right. Rotate the right foot forward 90 degrees to the left, the left foot 90 degrees to the left and the pelvis and torso to the left as you raise the right arm up over the head. Lower the left arm down to the side of the torso. Exhale, bend the left knee, extend the right heel slightly back behind the right toes, reaching the right arm forward and down to the left of the left knee. Place the palm of the right hand on the floor to the left of the left foot. Twist the torso to the left and reach the left arm forward and up over the head away from the right foot, with the palm of the hand facing down. Create a straight line with the body from the outside of the right foot to the left finger tips. Tilt the head back and look at the palm of the left hand--hasta drishti. Remain in Parivrtta Parshvakonasana on the left side for five deep breaths.

Inhale, raise the torso and straighten the left leg, as the right arm reaches forward, up and out to the right. Rotate the pelvis and torso to the right as you extend the left arm out to the left and rotate the left foot rotates forward so that it's parallel with the right foot. Exhale, hop the feet together 90 degrees to the left into Samastitihi and place the palms of the hands together into Anjali Mudra in front of the chest.

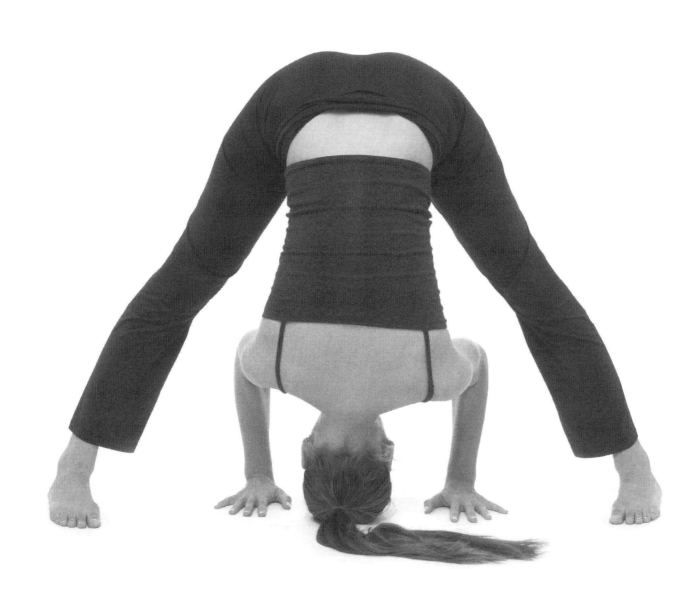

PRASARITA PADOTTANASANA A

Inhale, jump the feet three to four feet apart, 90 degrees to the right. Extend the arms out to the sides at shoulder height. Exhale, place the hands on the hips. Inhale, lift the ribcage. Exhale, fold the torso forward and place the palms of the hands shoulder width apart on the floor between the feet. Inhale, lift the head, until the arms and spine straighten. Exhale, bend the elbows back between the legs, keeping them shoulder width apart. Place the top of the head on the floor between the hands. Look toward the tip of the nose—nasa dristhti. Stay in Prasarita Padottanasana A for five breaths.

Inhale, lift the head until the arms and spine straighten, keeping the palms of the hands in contact with the floor. Exhale, place the hands on the hips. Inhale, raise the torso, with a straight spine, back up to standing and extend the arms out to the sides.

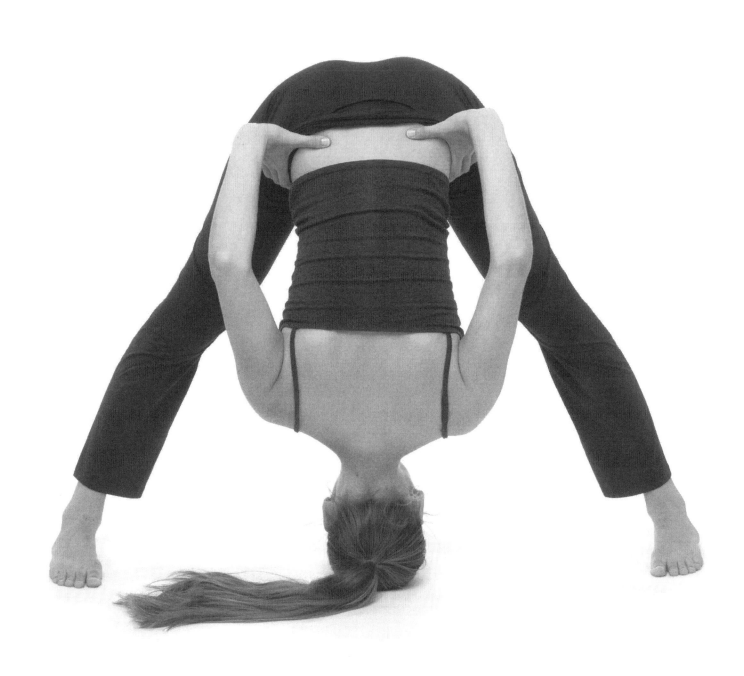

PRASARITA PADOTTANASANA B

Exhale, place the hands on the hips. Inhale, lift the ribcage. Exhale, fold the torso forward and down and place the top of the head on the floor between the feet. Keep the hands on the hips and look toward the tip of the nose—nasa drishti. Stay in Prasarita Padottanasana B for five breaths.

With one long inhale, lift the torso back up to standing and extend the arms out to the sides.

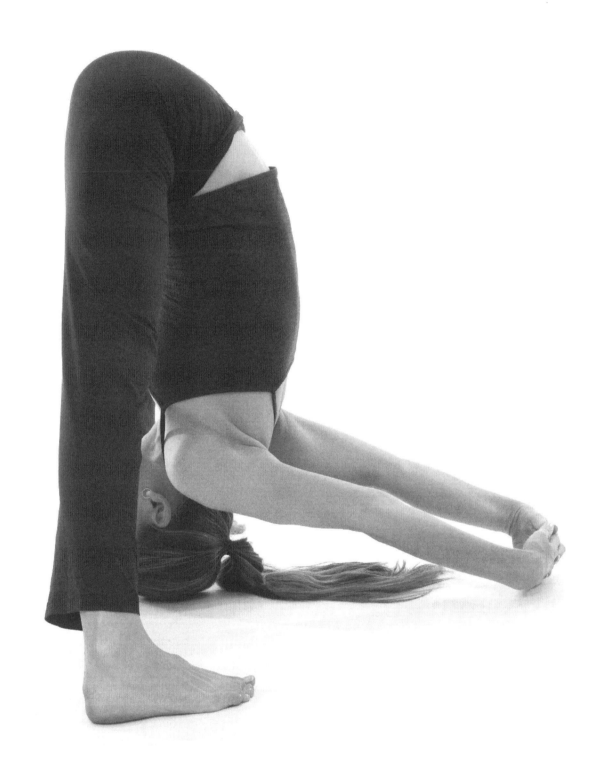

PRASARITA PADOTTANASANA C

Lower the arms, keeping them straight, and interlace the fingers behind the back. Inhale, lift the ribcage and pull the hands slightly down. Exhale, fold the torso forward and down, until the top of the head touches the floor between the feet as you reach the hands, keeping the arms straight, up and over the head until the fingers contact the floor. Look toward the tip of the nose–nasa drishti. Stay in Prasarita Padottanasana C for five breaths.

With one deep inhale, lift the arms and lower them down to the hips, raise the torso back up to standing and then extend the arms out to the sides at shoulder height.

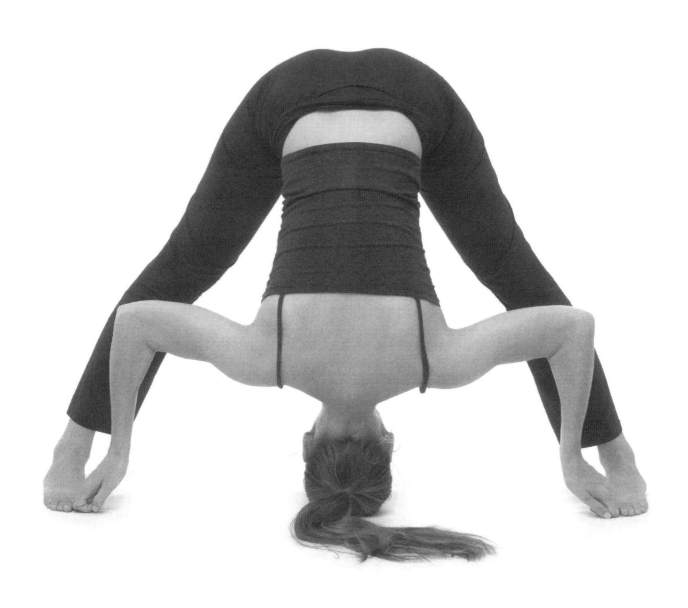

PRASARITA PADOTTANASANA D

Keeping the arms extended out to the sides, exhale and fold the torso forward. Reach toward the feet with the hands. Encircle the big toes with the first two fingers and thumbs. Inhale, lift the head, keeping hold of the big toes until the torso and arms straighten. Exhale, place the top of the head on the floor between the feet and lift the elbows up as the arms bend. Look towards the tip of the nose (Nasa Drishti) and take five deep breaths in this Prasarita Padottanasana D.

Inhale, lift the head, keeping hold of the toes until the arms and torso straighten. Exhale, place the hands on the hips. Inhale, raise the torso back up to standing and extend the arms out to the sides at shoulder height. Exhale, hop the hands and feet back together into Samastitihi.

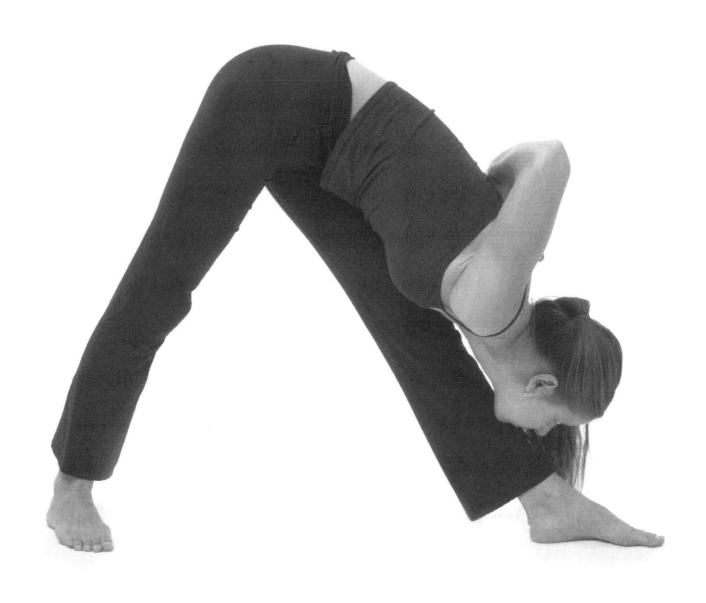

ASHTANGA YOGA

PARSHVOTTANASANA

Inhale, hop the feet three to four feet apart 90 degrees to the right and extend the arms out to the sides. Rotate the arms internally, bend the elbows and place the palms of the hands together behind the back between the shoulder blades, with the fingers pointing up. Rotate the right foot 90 degrees to the right and left foot 45 degrees to the right. Rotate the hips and torso to the right, by drawing the inner thighs together. Inhale, lift the ribcage and pull the elbows back. Exhale, fold the torso forward and down until it touches the right leg. Extend the chin forward, touch the chin to the shin and gaze toward the foot—pada drishti. Remain in Parshvottanasana on the right side for five breaths.

Inhale, lift the head and raise the torso back up to standing. Exhale, rotate the body to the left. Rotate the left foot 90 degrees to the left and the right foot 45 degrees to the left. Inhale lift the ribcage, pull the elbows back and press the palms together. Exhale, fold the torso forward until it touches the left leg, and reaching the chin forward, touch the chin to the shin and look toward the foot—pada drishti. Remain in Parshvottanasana on the left side for five breaths. Inhale, lift the head and raise the torso. Rotate to the right and extend the arms out to the sides. Exhale, hop the hands and feet back together into Samastitihi.

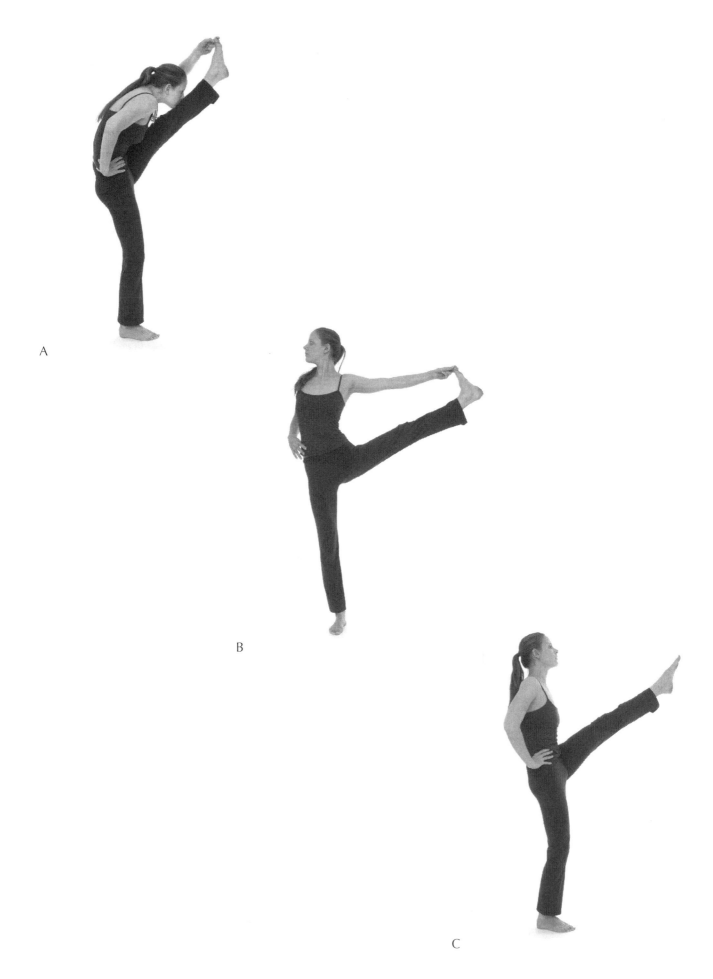

A

B

C

UTTHITA HASTA PADANGUSTASANA A, B & C

Place the left hand on the left hip. Raise the right leg, keeping it straight and encircle the right big toe with the first two fingers and thumb of the right hand. Keep both legs straight. Bend forward toward the right leg as you raise the leg up to touch the chin to the shin. Look toward the foot—pada drishti—and hold this asana (Uttitha Hasta Padangusthasana A) for five breaths. Inhale, raise the torso back up to standing and straighten the right arm. Then reach the right leg ninety degrees to the right and look to the left. This position (Uttitha Hasta Padangusthasana B) is held for five breaths. Exhaling, rotate the right leg back to the front and bend forward as you raise the leg up to touch the chin to the shin. Inhale, raise the torso back up to an upright position and release the grip around the right toe, and point the toes on the right foot. Place the right hand on the right hip. Keep the right leg raised for five breaths and look to the foot—pada drishti. Then place the right foot back down on the floor next to the left foot, into Samastitihi.

Place the right hand on the right hip. Raise the left leg and encircle the left big toe with the first two fingers and thumb of the left hand. Straighten both legs. Bend forward toward the left leg and raise the leg to touch chin to the shin. Look forward toward the foot—pada drishti—and hold this position for five breaths. Inhale, raise the torso back up to standing and straighten the left arm. Reach the left leg to the left and look to the right. Hold this position for five breaths. On the exhale reach the left leg back to the front and bend forward to touch the chin to the shin. Then raise the torso to an upright position and release the grip around the left toe. Point the left toes and place the left hand on the hip and look to the foot—pada drishti. Keep the left leg raised for five breaths. Then place the left foot on the floor next to the right foot, into Samastitihi.

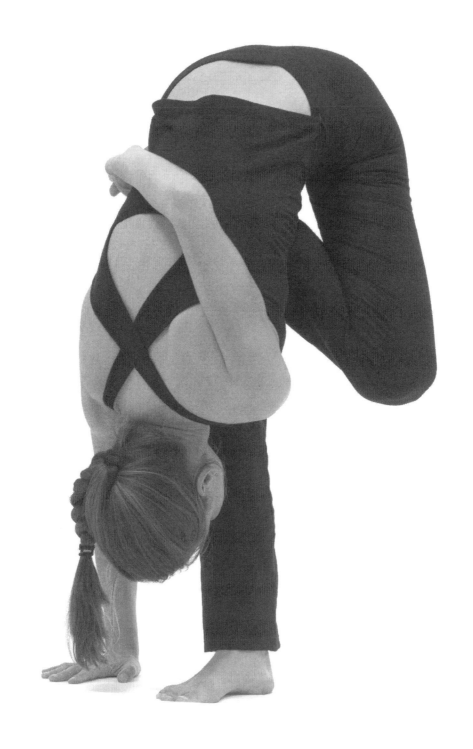

ASHTANGA YOGA

ARDHA BADDHA PADMOTTANASANA

Step into the left leg and lift the right foot up in front of the left leg, just below the hip on the inhale. Reach the right arm back and around the torso. Catch the right big toe from behind the back with the first two fingers of the right hand and encircle the big toe with the thumb. Place the left hand on the left hip, then exhale bend forward and place the left hand on the floor to the left of the left foot. Inhale lift the head until the left arm straightens. Exhale, reach the chin forward and down until it touches the shin of the left leg. Look toward the foot—pada drishti. Remain in this asana for five breaths. Inhale lift the head until the left arm and the torso straighten. Exhale, place the left hand on the left hip. Inhale, lift the head and raise the torso back up to standing. Release the grip around the right big toe and place the right foot down on the floor next to the left foot.

Shift the weight into the right foot and lift the left foot, placing it in front of the right leg just below the hip. Reach the left arm back and around the torso to the right. Catch the left big toe from behind the back with the first two fingers of the left hand and encircle the big toe with the thumb. Place the right hand on the right hip. Exhale, fold the torso forward and down and place the right hand on the floor to the right of the right foot. Inhale, lift the head, until the right arm and the torso straighten. Exhale, draw the torso in toward the right leg and extend the chin forward until it touches the shin. Look toward the right foot—pada drishti. Remain in the asana for five breaths. Inhale, raise the head until the right arm and the torso straighten. Exhale, place the right hand on the right hip. Inhale, raise the torso back up to standing. Release the grasp of the left hand on the left foot and place the left foot on the floor next to the right foot, into Samastitihi.

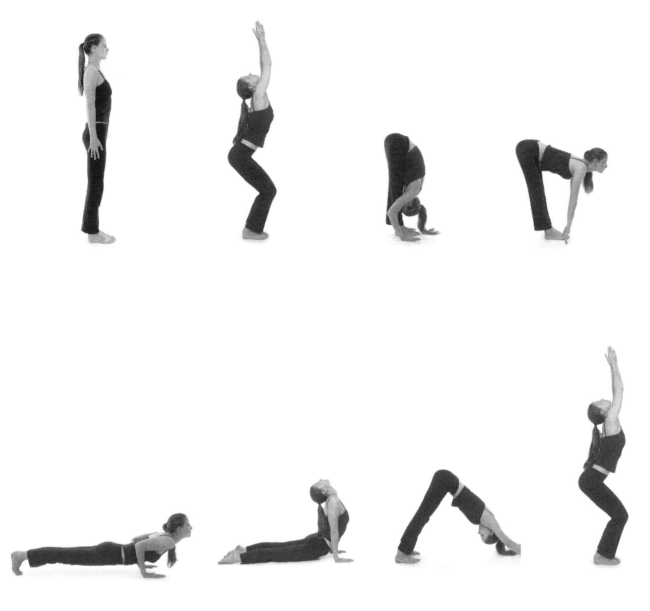

UTKATASANA

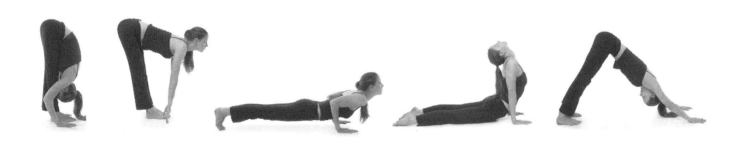

WARRIOR SEQUENCE

To transition from the standing asanas to the seated asanas of the primary series, practice the asanas of Surya Namaskara A until Adho Mukha Shvanasana. Stay in Adho Mukha Shvanasana for only one breath and jump forward between the hands, bend the knees and reach the arms up and over the head into Utkatasana for five breaths. At the end of the fifth inhale, reach the arms out and down next to the feet and straighten the legs into Uttanasana. Inhale, lift the head and straighten the spine. Exhale hop back into Chaturanga Dandasana. Inhale, draw the chest forward and up into Urdhva Mukha Shvanasana. Exhale, lift the hips back and up into Adho Mukha Shvanasana. Rotate the left foot out 45 degrees, and step the right foot forward between the hands. Bend the right knee and reach the arms out and up into Virabhadrasana A. Remain in this asana for five breaths.

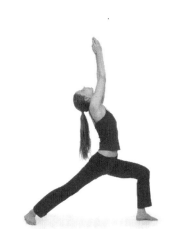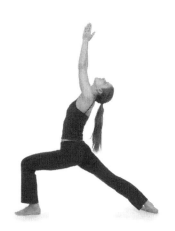

A

VIRABHADRASANA

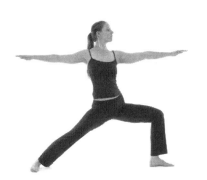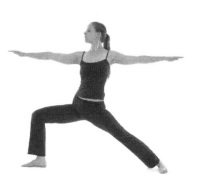

B

VIRABHADRASANA

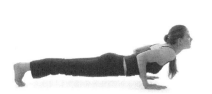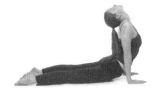

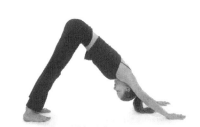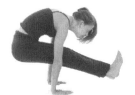

WARRIOR SEQUENCE

Inhale, straighten the right leg and rotate one hundred and eighty degrees to the left. Bend the left leg into Virabhadrasana A on the left side. Remain in this asana for five breaths. After completing the fifth inhale, exhale into Virabhadrasana B on the left side by rotating the hips to the right, rotating the right foot slightly to the right and reaching the arms out to the sides, at shoulder level, parallel to the floor, above the legs. Turn the head to the left. The palms of the hands face down, the fingers are straight and together. Direct the gaze to the left hand—hasta drishti. Stay in this asana for 5 breaths. Inhale, straighten the left leg and rotate the left foot 90 degrees to the right. Turn the head and the right foot to the right and bend the right leg on

the exhale. The arms remain in the same position and the gaze is shifted to the right hand—hasta drishti. Stay in Virabhadrasana B on the right for five breaths. On the exhale reach the left arm down to the floor to the left of the right foot. Place the right hand on the floor, to the right of the right foot and step the right foot back next to the left foot as the arms bend into Chaturanga Dandasana. Reach the chin forward and direct the gaze to the nose—nasa drishti. Inhale, reach the chest forward and up into Urdhva Mukha Shvanasana. Exhale lift the hips, back and up into Adho Mukha Shvanasana. From here, bend the knees slightly and hop the feet through the arms into a seated position, with straight legs. Inhale, lift the chest and straighten the spine.

PRIMARY SERIES

The Primary Series is referred to as Yoga Chikitsa. Yoga Chikitsa

is translated as Yoga Therapy. It is the method by which disease is

eliminated from the body, through practicing this specific sequence

of Yoga Asanas. The Asanas, which are unique to the Primary Series,

stimulate Apana Vayu, the exhaling breath as well as the downward

moving energy in the body. This produces a calming effect and

stimulates the elimination of toxins from the body.

Practicing the Primary Series facilitates overcoming addictions. When

adjusting your life to practicing the Primary Series five or six times a

week, it is important to simultaneously adjust your lifestyle to include a

healthy vegetarian diet and sufficient rest.

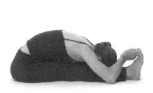
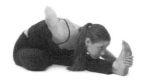
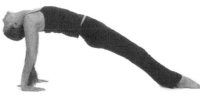
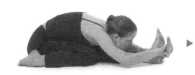

PASCHIMOTTANASANA

PURVOTTANASANA

ARDHA BADDHA PADMA
PASCHIMOTTANASANA

TIRYANG MUKHA EKA PADA
PASCHIMOTTANASANA

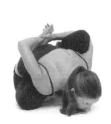
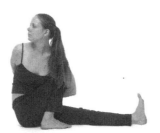
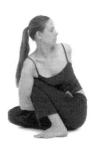
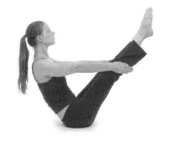

B

C
MARICHYASANA

D

NAVASANA

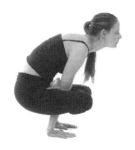
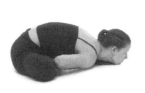
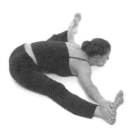
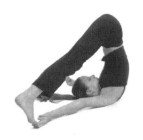

KUKKUTASANA

BADDHA KONASANA

UPAVISTHA
KONASANA

SUPTA KONASANA

PRIMARY SERIES

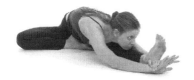
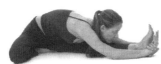
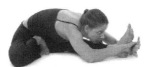
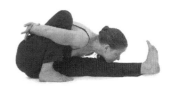

A

B

C

A

JANU SHIRSASANA

MARICHYASANA

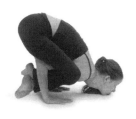
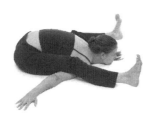
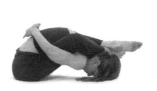
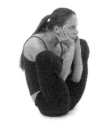

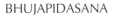

BHUJAPIDASANA

KURMASANA

SUPTA.KURMASANA

GARBHA PINDASANA

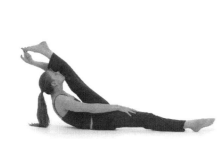
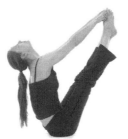
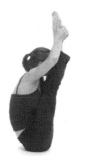
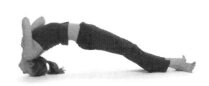

SUPTA
PADANGUSTASANA

UBHAYA
PADANGUSTASANA

URDHVA MUKHA
PASCHIMOTTANASANA

SETU BANDHASANA

Paschimottanasana is foremost among asanas.
It reverses the breaths flow, kindles the digestive fire,
flattens the belly and brings good health.

Quote: Hatha Yoga Pradipika – Chapter 1, Verse 29

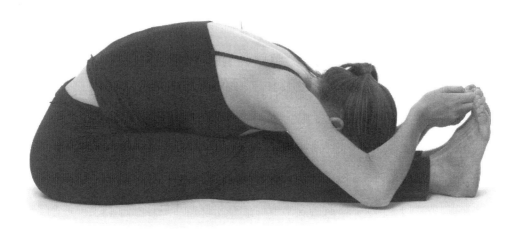

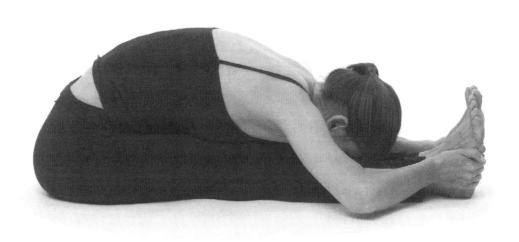

PASCHIMOTTANASANA A & B

Sit with a straight spine, the legs together and feet flexed in Dandasana. Exhale and reach forward to encircle the big toes with the first two fingers and thumbs of each hand. Inhale, straighten the spine, by lifting the head and chest until the arms straighten. Exhale, pull forward by bending the elbows, and reach the chest and chin forward and down until the chest touches the legs. Look forward to the feet—pada drishti. Remain in Paschimottanasana A for five breaths.

Then, inhale lift the head and chest until the arms straighten. Change the hand position from encircling the big toes to holding the sides of the feet. Exhale, pull forward and down with the arms, engage the abdomen and draw the chest forward and down to the legs. Reach the chin forward and look toward the feet—pada drishti. Stay in Paschimottanasana B for five breaths.

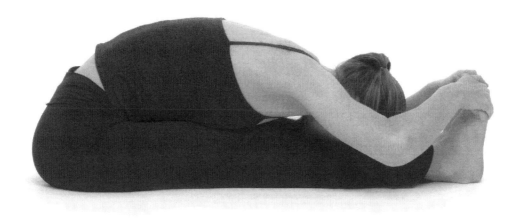

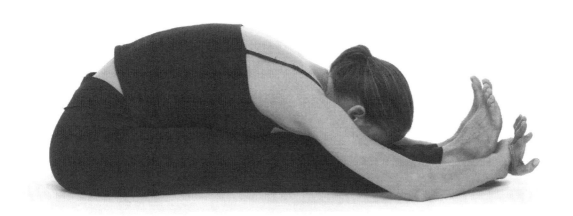

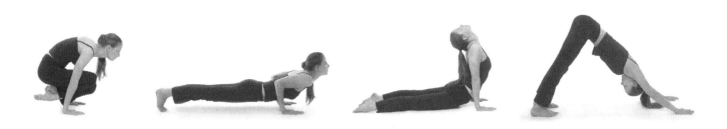

ASHTANGA YOGA

PASCHIMOTTANASANA C & D

Inhale, lift the head and chest until the arms straighten and change the hand position from holding the outsides of the feet to reaching over the toes. Place the palms of the hands on the soles of the feet. On the exhale, pull forward and down with the arms. Reach the chest forward and down to the legs, extend the chin forward, and look toward the feet—pada drishti. Keep the legs straight and engage the abdominal muscles to deepen the forward bend. Remain in Paschimottanasana C for five deep breaths.

vInhale, lift the head and chest until the arms straighten. Change the hand position from reaching over the tops of the feet to reaching around the outsides of the feet with both hands, with the palms of the hands facing forward and take hold of one wrist. Then, on the exhaling breath, bend the arms to reach the chest forward and down to the legs. Extend the chin forward and look toward the feet—pada drishti. Remain in Paschimottanasa D for five breaths.

Inhale, lift the head and raise the torso until the arms straighten. Release the hands, raise the torso to an upright position. Place the hands on the floor next to the hips. Exhale, press into the arms and engage the abdominal muscles to lift the hips and the legs off the floor and swing them through the arms and extend them back into Chaturanga Dandasana. Inhale, reach the chest forward and up into Urdhva Mukha Shvanasana. Exhale, lift the hips into Adho Mukha Shvanasana. Bend the knees and jump through the arms, extending the legs forward into Dandasana.

Once the chest lays comfortably on the legs in Paschimottansana, one may eliminate Paschimottanasana B (holding the sides of the feet) and C (reaching over the feet with the hands) and practice only Paschimottanasana A (encircling the big toes with the fingers) and D (reaching around the feet and clasping the left wrist with the right hand).

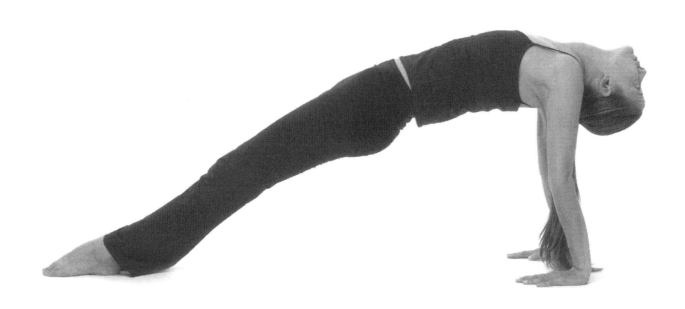

PURVOTTANASANA

Place the hands on the floor about one foot behind the hips, with the fingers pointing forward in the direction of the feet. Keeping the arms straight, on the inhale, lift the hips by pressing the heels of the feet into the floor with straight legs. Point the toes and press the soles of the feet into the floor. Tilt the head back by reaching the chin up and back and look toward the nose—nasa drishti. Remain in Purvottanasana for five breaths.

Exhale, place the hips back onto the floor. Place the hands next to the hips. Inhale, lift the hips and legs and swing them back into Chaturanga Dandasana. Inhale into Urdhva Mukha Shvanasana. Exhale into Adho Mukha Shvanasana and jump through the arms. Sit in Dandanasana with the legs extended forward.

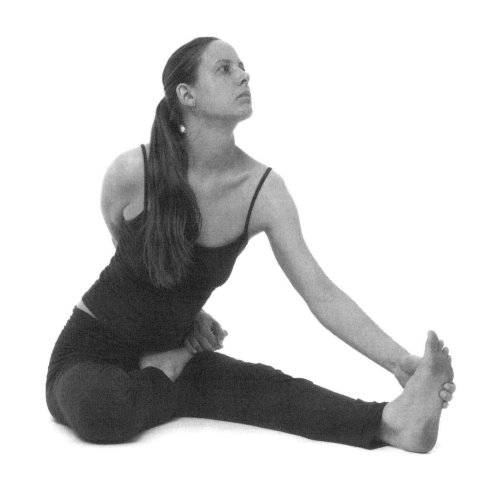

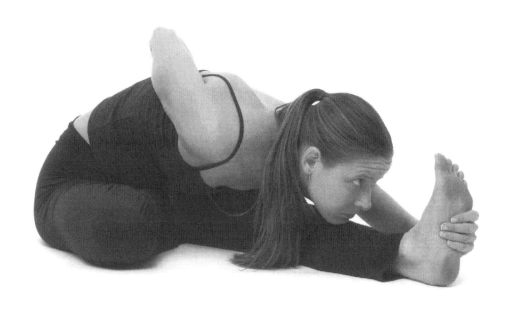

ARDHA BADDHA PADMA PASCHIMOTTANASANA

Place the right foot into the crease of the left hip and lower the right knee to the floor. Reach the right arm behind the back and encircle the right big toe with the first two fingers and the thumb of the right hand. Straighten the left leg and flex the left foot. Reach forward with the left hand and hold the outside of the left foot. Inhale and lift the head and chest until the left arm straightens. Exhale, pull the chest forward with the left arm until it touches the left leg. Reach the chin forward and look toward the left foot—pada drishti. Remain in Ardha Baddha Padma Paschimottanasana on the right side for five breaths.

Inhale, lift the head and torso, until the left arm straightens. Release the hands, extend the right leg and place the palms of the hands on the floor on either side of the hips. Exhale, lift the hips and legs and swing them back, through the arms, into Chaturanga Dandasana. Inhale into Urdhva Mukha Shvanasana. Exhale into Adho Mukha Shvanasana and jump back through the arms. Straighten the legs.

Then, place the left foot into the crease of the right hip and enter Ardha Baddha Padma Paschimottanasana on the left side. Hold the asana for five breaths. Exit the asana on the inhale and swing back into Chaturanga Dandanasa on the exhale. Complete the vinyasa and return to a seated position with straight legs.

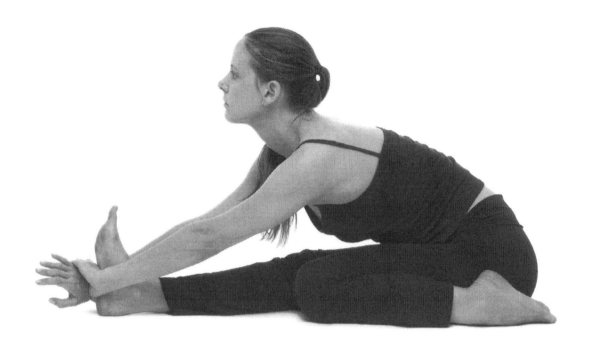

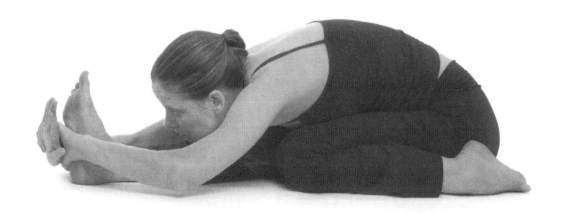

TIRYANG MUKHA EKA PADA PASCHIMOTTANSANA

Shift your weight into the left hip, bend the right leg and fold the knee completely, placing the top of right foot on the floor next to the right hip. The sole of the foot faces up, and the toes point back. Then shift the weight back into the right hip and draw the right leg in next to the left leg until the knees touch. Reach the arms forward and with the palms of the hands facing forward, take hold of one wrist around the left foot. Inhale, lift the head and chest until the spine and arms straighten. Exhale, pull the chest forward and down with the arms until the chest touches the left leg. Reach the chin forward, placing it on the left shin, and look toward the left foot—pada drishti. Remain in Tiryang Mukha Eka Pada Paschimottansana on the right side for five deep breaths.

Inhale, lift the head and chest until the arms straighten. Release the hands and raise the torso into an upright position. Extend the right leg forward next to the left leg. Press the palms of the hands into the floor next to the hips. Exhale, lift the hips and legs and swing them back, through the arms, into Chaturanga Dandasana. Complete the vinyasa and hop forward through the arms. Straighten the legs in preparation for Tiryang Mukha Eka Pada Paschimottansana on the left side.

Shift the weight into the right hip, bend the left leg and place the top of the left foot next to the left hip, with the sole of the foot facing up and the toes pointing back. Then, enter Tiryang Mukha Eka Pada Paschimottansana on the left side and remain in the asana for five deep breaths. Inhale, raise the head and chest. Exhale into Chaturanga Dandanasa. Inhale into Urdhva Mukha Shvanasana. Exhale into Adho Mukha Shvanasana, and hop through the arms back to seated with the legs straight and together and the feet flexed.

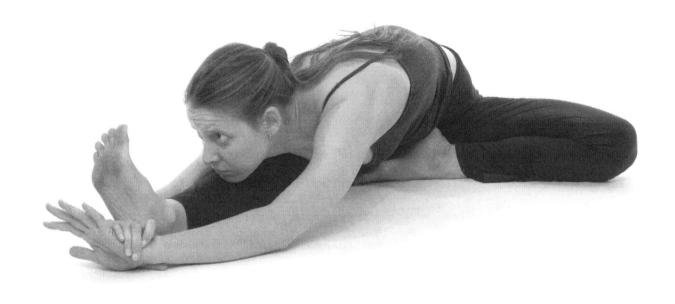

JANUSHIRSHASANA A

Bend the right leg and fold the knee completely by drawing the right heel in close to the right hip. Place the right knee on the floor to the right. Extend the right knee back until you create a 135 degree angle between the left leg and the right thigh. Straighten the left leg straight, by pressing the left thigh into the floor. Flex the left foot. Reach the arms forward and, with the palms facing forward, take hold of one wrist around the left foot. Inhale lift the head and draw the chest forward toward the left foot. Exhale, reach the chest forward and down until it touches the left leg. Reach the chin forward onto the left shin and look toward the left foot—pada drishti. Remain in Janushirshasana A on the right side for five deep breaths. Eventually, the toes on the right foot point and the top of the right foot and ankle press into the floor as the right knee reaches back 135 degrees.

Inhale, lift the head and raise the torso, until the arms straighten. Release the hands and extend the right leg forward next to the left leg. Place the hands on the floor next to the hips and press into the hands. Lift the hips and legs and swing them back into Chaturanga Dandasana on the exhale. Inhale, reach the chest forward and up and tilt the head back into Urdhva Mukha Shvanasana. Exhale, lift the hips back and up. Reach the heels back and down into the floor, and draw the chin into the chest for Adho Mukha Shvanasana. Then, lifting the hips slightly, hop through the arms with straight legs into an upright seated position.

Then enter Janushirshasana A on the left side by bending the left leg and drawing the left heel in close to the left hip. Drop the left knee down to the floor to the left and reach the left knee back as you reach forward with the arms, with palms facing forward, and take hold of one wrist around the right foot. Inhale, lift the chest and extend the right leg by pressing the right thigh into the floor. Exhale, reach the chest forward and down until it touches the right leg, and extend the chin forward on the right shin. Look toward the right foot—pada drishti. Remain in Janushirshasana A on the left side for five breaths. Inhale, lift the head and chest until the arms straighten. Release the hands and raise the torso into an upright position. Exhale swing back into Chaturanga Dandasana. Inhale into Urdhva Mukha Shvanasana and exhale into Adho Mukha Shvanasana. Hop through the arms and extend the legs forward.

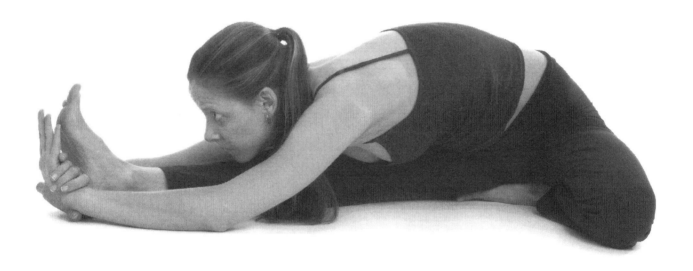

JANUSHIRSHASANA B

Enter Janushirshasana B on the right side, by bending the right leg and folding the knee completely, by drawing the right heel in close to the public bone. Drop the right knee down onto the floor to the right. Extend the knee to the side, until the right thigh is at a 90 degree angle to the left leg. Flex the right foot so that the right toes point in the direction of the left foot. Then, lift the hips and sit on the right foot so that the heel of the right foot presses into the floor of the pelvis between the sit bones. Extend into the left leg and flex the left foot. Reach forward with the arms and with palms facing forward, take hold of one wrist around the left foot. Inhale lift the head and chest until the arms straighten, and exhale, reach the chest forward and down onto the left leg. Extend the chin forward on the left shin and look toward the left foot—pada drishti. Stay in Janushirshasana B for five breaths. Then, inhale raise the head and chest until the arms straighten. Unclasp the hands, raise the torso into an upright position, and lift the hips up and back off the right foot. Extend the right leg forward next to the left leg. Exhale into Chaturanga Dandanasa. Inhale into Urdhva Mukha Shvanasana, and exhale into Adho Mukha Shvanasana. Hop forward through the arms, into a seated position with straight legs.

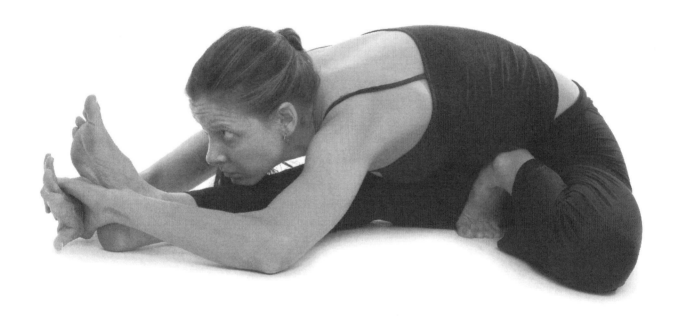

JANUSHIRSHASANA C

Bend the right leg and draw the right heel in close to public bone. Drop the right knee down to the right. Reach underneath the right leg just above the right ankle with the right hand and clasp the right lower leg with the palm of the right hand. Rotate the lower right leg externally with the right hand and flex the feet and toes. Place the toes on the floor to the left of the upper left thigh, close to the public bone. Raise the right heel, until the foot is perpendicular to the floor up and the arch of the right foot touches the inside of the left thigh. Keep the right hip in contact with the floor and reach the knee down to the floor at a forty-five degree angle to the left leg. Reach forward and take hold of one wrist around the left foot, with the palms of the hands facing forward. Inhale, lift the head and chest until the arms straighten. Exhale,

reach the chest forward and down onto the left leg, extend the chin forward onto the left shin and look to the left foot (Pada Drishti). Remain in Janushirshasana C for five breaths. Inhale, lift the head and chest until the arms straighten. Unclasp the hands and raise the torso into an upright position. Extend the right leg forward next to the left leg. Exhale swing back into Chaturanga Dandasana. Inhale into Urdhva Mukha Shvanasana and exhale into Adho Mukha Shvanasana. Hop forward through the arms into a seated position with straight legs.

Then, enter Janushirshasana C on the left side. Remain in the asana for five breaths. Exit the asana on the inhale and then move through a vinyasa back to a seated position.

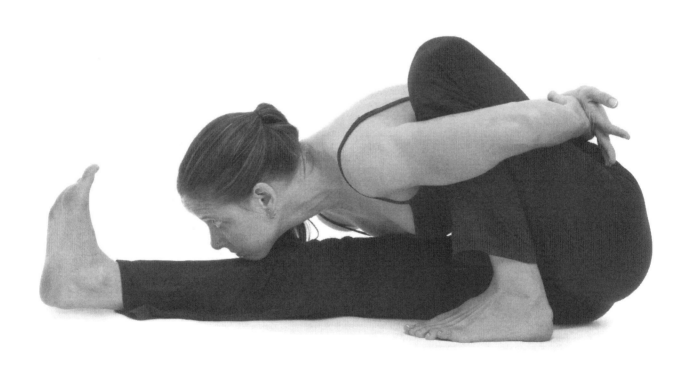

MARICHYASANA A

Extend the left leg forward. Bend the right leg, into a squatting position, with the right foot on the floor in front of the right hip. Reach the right arm forward and to the left of the right leg. Rotate the right arm internally and wrap it back and around the bent right leg and torso. Simultaneously reach the left arm back behind the torso to meet the right hand. Take hold of one wrist with the palms of the hands facing out. Inhale and lift the head and chest. Exhale and reach the chest forward and down onto the left leg, extending the chin forward onto the shin. Look toward the left foot—pada drishti. Press the left thigh into the floor and flex the left foot. Remain in Marichyasana A for five breaths. Inhale, lift the head and chest. Release the arms. Exhale, press the hands into the floor and swing back into Chaturanga Dandasana. Inhale into Urdhva Mukha Shvanasana. Exhale into Adho Mukha Shvanasana. Hop forward through the arms.

Enter Marichyasana A on the left side by bending the left leg into a squatting position and wrapping the arms around the bent left leg and torso. Inhale and lift the chest, and exhale, bending forward onto the right leg. Remain in Marichyasana A on the left side for five breaths. Inhale, raise the head and chest. Release the arms. Exhale, into Chaturanga Dandasana. Inhale into Urdhva Mukha Shvanasana. Exhale into Adho Mukha Shvanasana. Jump through and sit down with the legs together and extended forward.

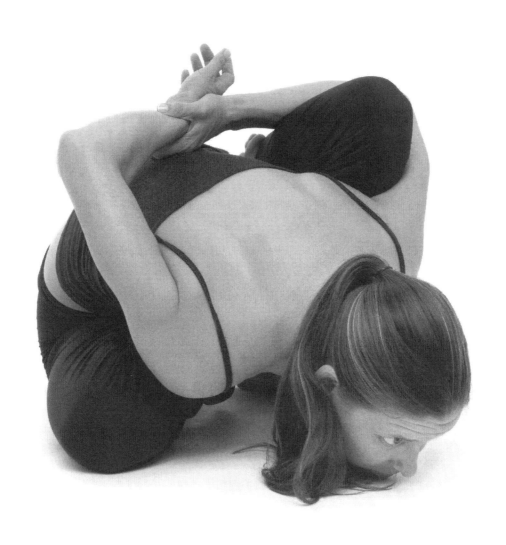

MARICHYASANA B

Bend the left leg and place the outside of left foot, above the right thigh, into the crease of the right hip. Press the left knee into the floor to the left. Shift your weight into the left hip and bend the right leg into a squatting position. The right hip will naturally lift slightly off of the floor. Then, wrap the right arm back and around the right leg and torso. Reach the left arm behind the torso and take hold of one wrist with the palms of the hands facing out. Inhale, lift the head and chest. Exhale and fold the torso forward between the left knee and the right foot. Place the chin on the floor. Look softly toward the tip of the nose—nasa drishti. Hold Marichyasana B on the right side for five breaths. Inhale, raise the head and chest. Release the arms, raise the torso and extend first the right leg out and then the left leg forward next to the right leg. Exhale swing back into Chaturanga Dandasana. Inhale and reach the chest forward and up into Urdhva Mukha Shvanasana. Exhale and lift the hips up into Adho Mukha Shvanasana. Jump through and sit down with the legs extended forward in front of you.

Enter Marichyasana B on the right side by bending the right leg and placing the right foot above the left thigh into the crease of the right hip. Press the right knee on the floor and place the left foot on floor into a squatting position. The left hip will naturally lift slightly off the floor. Reach around and take hold of one wrist behind the torso. Inhale, and lift the head and chest. Fold the torso forward on the exhale and hold this position for five breaths. Inhale, raise the head and chest. Release the arms and extend first the left leg forward and then the right leg forward. Exhale and swing back into Chaturanga Dandasana. Inhale and reach the chest forward and up into Urdhva Mukha Shvanasana. Exhale and lift the hips up into Adho Mukha Shvanasana. Jump through and sit down with the legs extended forward.

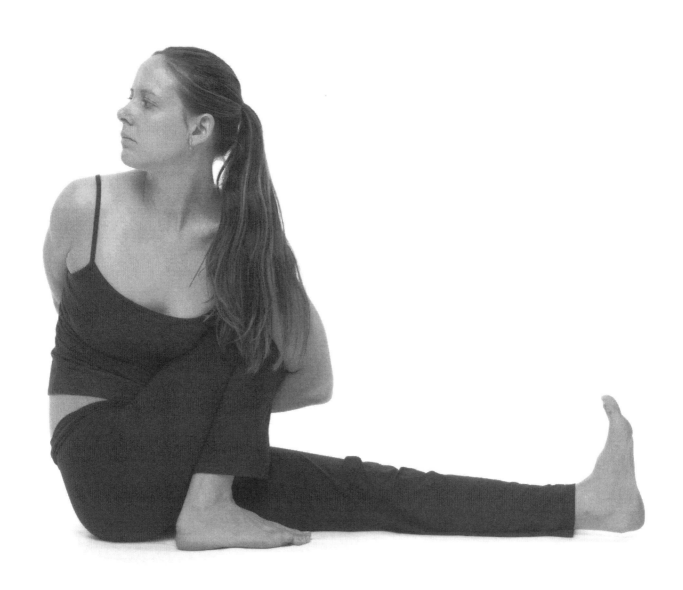

MARICHYASANA C

Bend the right leg and place the right foot on the floor into a squatting position. The right hip naturally lifts slightly up off of the floor. Place the right hand on the floor behind you. Raise the left arm on the inhaling breath. Then, on the exhale, twist the torso to the right, bending the left elbow as you lower the left arm down to the right of the right bent leg. Reach the left arm to the left and wrap it around the right leg and torso. Lift the right hand and reach it to the right and back around the torso to meet the left hand. Clasp the right wrist with the left hand. Twist the head to the right and look to the right—parshva drishti. Extend and activate the left leg, by pressing the left thigh into the floor and flexing the left foot. Remain in Marchiyasana C on the right side for five breaths. Inhale and release the hands, rotating the torso to the left. Extend the right leg forward next to the left leg. Exhale into Chaturanga Dandasana. Inhale into Urdhva Mukha Shvanasana. Exhale into Adho Mukha Shvanasana and jump through to sitting down with the legs together extended forward.

Enter Marichyasana C on the left side by bending the left leg and twisting the torso to the left. Wrap the arms around the bent left leg and the torso, clasping the left wrist with the right hand. Rotate the head to the left. Look to the left—parshva drishti. Remain in Marichyasana C for five breaths. Inhale and release the arms, twisting the torso back to the right. Extend the left leg forward next to the right leg. Exhale into Chaturanga Dandasana. Inhale into Urdhva Mukha Shvanasana. Exhale into Adho Mukha Shvanasana. Jump through and sit down with the legs straight and extended forward.

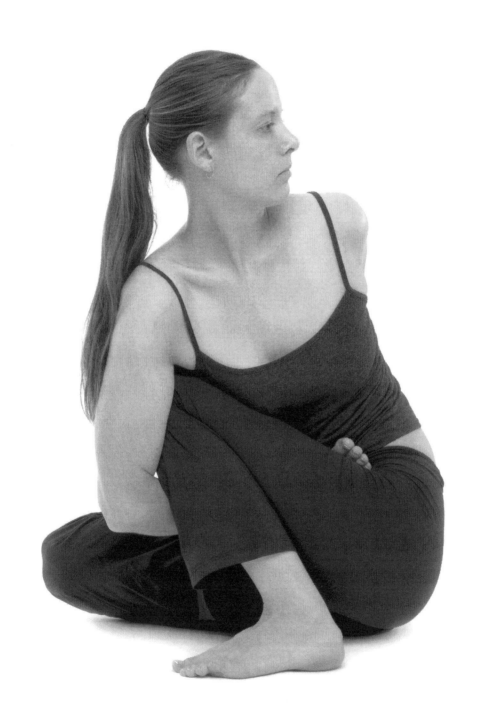

ASHTANGA YOGA

MARICHYASANA D

Bend the left leg and place the left foot in the crease of the right hip above the thigh. Press the left outer thigh into the floor and bend the right leg into a squatting position. The right hip will naturally lift slightly off of the floor. Inhale and raise the left arm, placing the palm of the right hand on the floor behind you for support. On the exhale, twist to the right as you bend the left arm, and lower the left elbow down to the outside of the left thigh. Straighten and rotate the left arm internally, then wrap the left arm around the left leg and the torso to the left. Lift the right hand and reach behind the torso to clasp the left wrist with the right hand. Twist the head to the right and look to the right—parshva drishti. Remain in Marichyasana D on the right side for five breaths.

Inhale and release the arms, straightening the right leg and extending the left leg forward next to the right leg. Exhale and lift the hips and legs, swinging back into Chaturanga Dandasana. Inhale into Urdhva Mukha Shvanasana and exhale into Adho Mukha Shvanasana. Jump through the arms and sit down.

Then enter Marichyasana D on the left side by bending the right leg and placing the right foot in the crease of the left hip above the thigh. Press the right knee into the floor and shift your weight into your right hip. Bend the left leg and place the left foot on the floor with the heel of the left foot close to the left hip, which lifts slightly up off of the floor. Twist to the left and wrap the arms around the left leg and torso. Clasp the right wrist with the left hand. Twist the head to the left and look to the left—parshva drishti. Stay in Marichyasana D on the left side for five breaths. Release the arms and extend the legs. Exhale back into Chaturanga Dandasana. Inhale into Urdhva Mukha Shvanasana and exhale into Adho Mukha Shvanasana.

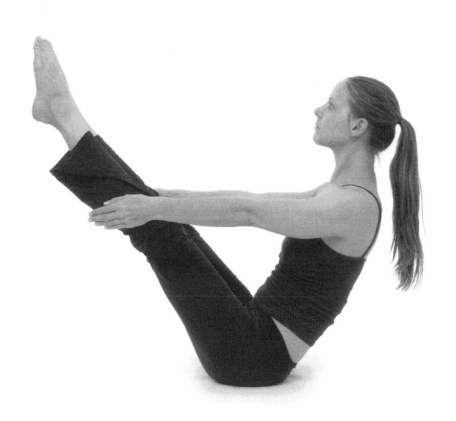

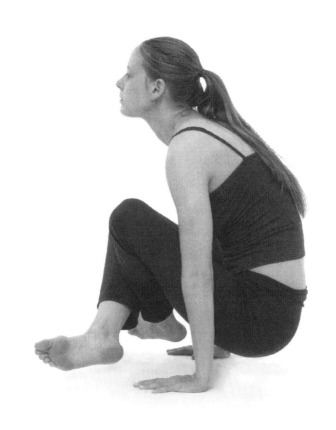

NAVASANA

From Adho Mukha Shvanasana, jump through the arms and raise the legs straight and together, about 45 degrees off of the floor, as you lean back 45 degrees with a straight spine. Point the toes. Straighten the arms and raise them parallel to each other until they're parallel to the floor. Rotate the arms so that the palms of the hands face each other. Look toward the feet—pada drishti. Stay here for five breaths.

Place the palms of the hands on the floor next to the hips. Bend the knees and cross the ankles and lift the hips and legs on the inhale. Exhale and place the hips back on the floor. Enter Navasana again for five breaths. Repeat the lift and enter Navasana three more times. Navasana is entered and held for five breaths five times. Then lift up and swing back into Chaturanga Dandasana. Inhale Urdhva Mukha Shvanasana. Exhale Adho Mukha Shvanasana.

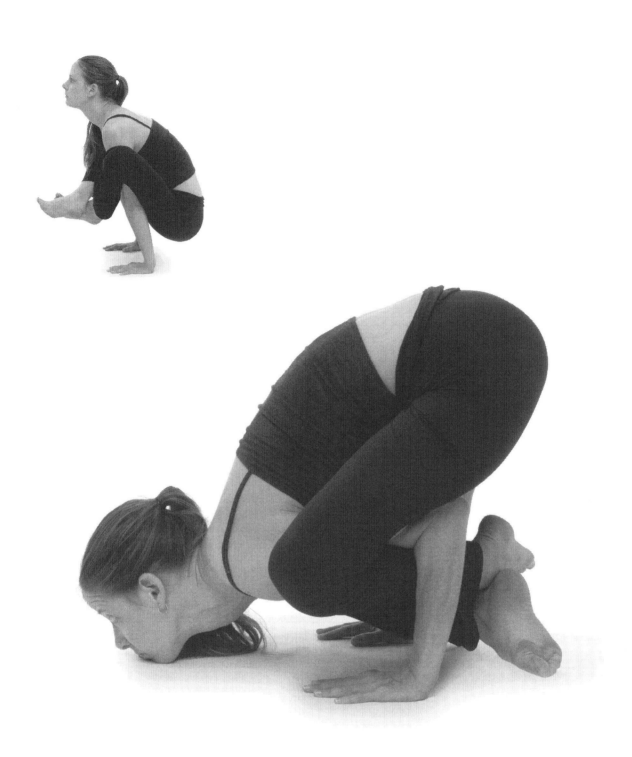

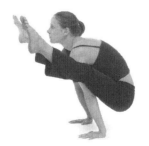

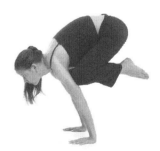

BUJA PIDASANA

Enter Buja Pidasana from Adho Mukha Shvanasana by jumping the feet around the arms. Keep the arms straight and the hands shoulder width apart. Place the inner thighs high on the upper arms and drop the weight of the body into the hands. Lift the legs and cross the right foot over the left foot in front of the arms. Bend the elbows and shift the weight forward, until the head touches the floor as you swing the feet back through the arms. Point the toes back. At first, the crown of the head is placed on the floor and eventually the chin is placed on the floor. Look toward the nose—nasa drishti--and stay here for five breaths.

Inhale and lift the head, straighten the arms and swing the legs forward through the arms. Uncross the feet and straighten the legs forward and up at a 45 degree angle. Point the toes into Tittibhasana. Exhale and bend the knees, shifting your weight forward. Swing the legs back so the shins rest on the upper arms and the toes touch. Straighten the arms, lift the feet and point the toes back into Bakasana. Then lift the hips slightly and extend the legs back into Chaturanga Dandasana. Inhale into Urdhva Mukha Shvanasana. Exhale into Adho Mukha Shvanasana.

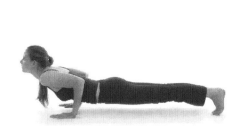 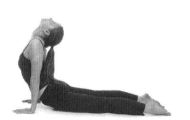 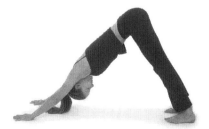

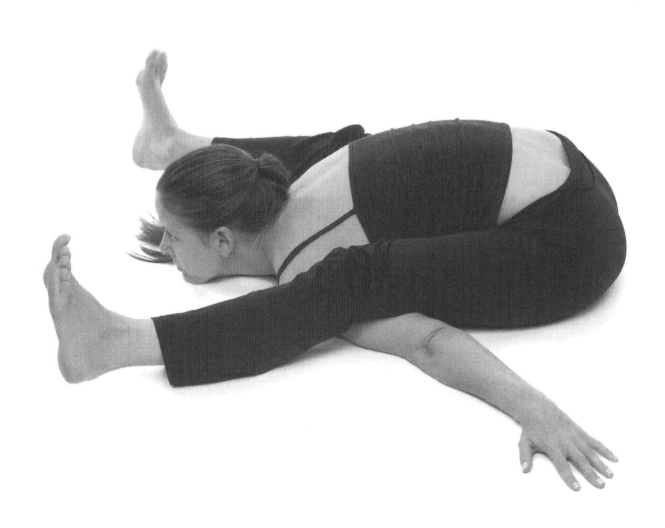

KURMASANA

From Adho Mukha Shvanasana, jump around the arms again.
Then sit down and reach the arms back, under the legs, along
the floor with the palms of the hands facing down. Straighten
the legs and flex the feet, until the heels lift off of the floor, as
the torso lowers down to the floor until the chest presses gently
into the floor. Reach the chin forward and set the gaze toward
the tip of the nose—nasa drishti. Stay here in Kurmasana for
five deep breaths.

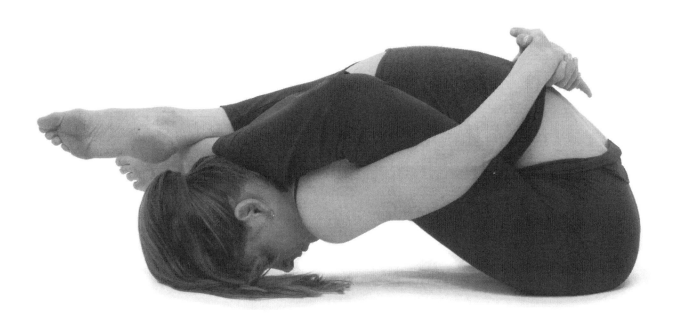

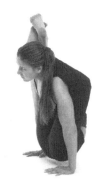 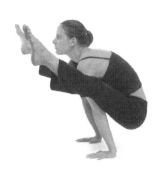 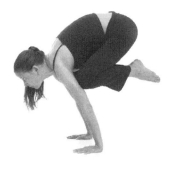

SUPTA KURMASANA

Then, bend the knees slightly and place the forehead on the floor. Reach the arms back and around the legs and torso. Clasp one wrist behind the back. Rotate the thighs externally and cross the right foot over the left foot above the head. Stay here in Supta Kurmasana for five breaths.

Release the hands and place the palms of the hands on the floor underneath the shoulders. Keep the feet crossed behind the head and lift the head and legs up off of the floor, by straightening the arms. Press into the hands and lift the hips up off of the floor. Then straighten the legs into Tittibhasana. Exhale and swing the legs back into Bakasana. Hop back into Chaturanga Dandasana. Complete the vinyasa, jump through and sit down.

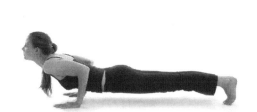 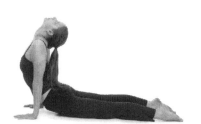 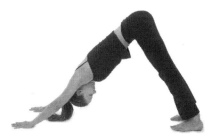

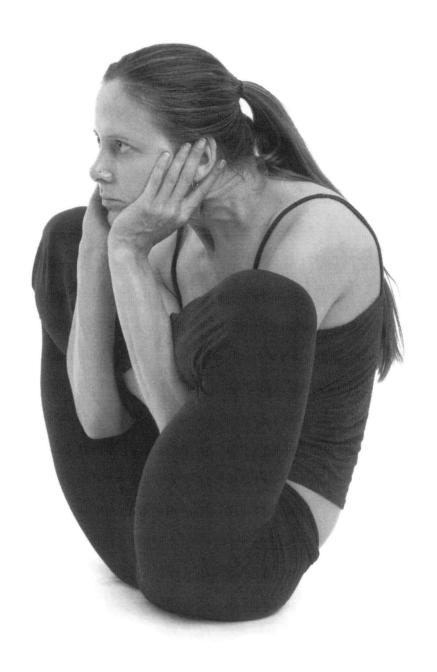

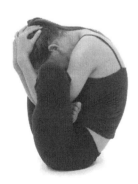
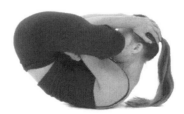
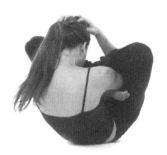

ASHTANGA YOGA

Settle in Padmasana. Reach the hands between the knees and thighs. Place the hands on the earth. Lift into the sky. This is Kukkutasana.

Hatha Yoga Pradipika – Chapter 1, Verse 23

GARBHA PINDASANA

Enter Padamasana by bending the right leg and placing the right foot into the crease of the left hip above the thigh. Then drop the right knee to the floor and bend the left leg, placing the left foot into the crease of the right hip above the thigh as the left knee drops to the floor. Lift the knees and reach the right arm through the legs in the space below the right knee and above the left lower leg. Then reach the left arm through the legs in the space below the left knee and above the right lower leg. Extend the arms completely through the legs until the elbows extend out beyond the legs. Then, bend the elbows to lift the hands up to the face. Hold the face with the hands and balance on the hips. Stay here for five breaths. Lower the chin down to the chest and place the hands on the top of the head. Rock back toward the shoulders on the exhale and rock up toward the hips on the inhale, five times, in a clock-wise circle, until you again face forward.

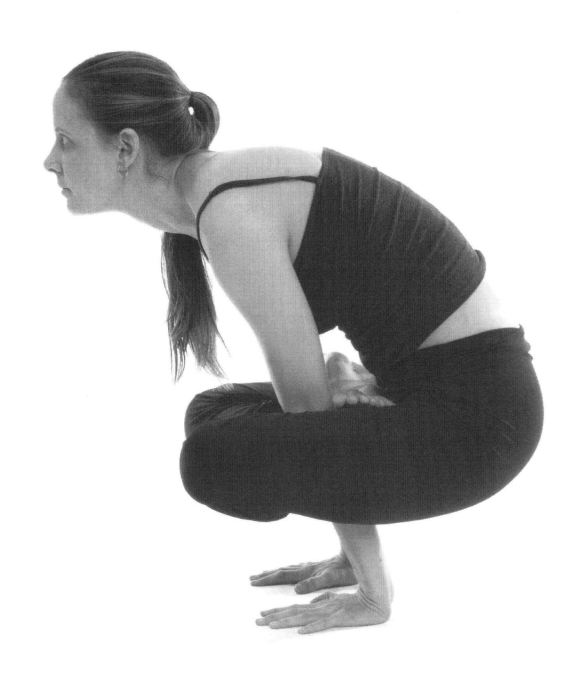

ASHTANGA YOGA

KUKKUTASANA

During the last forward rock in Garbha Pindasana, release the hands from the head. Straighten the arms and rock up to press the palms of the hands into the floor and lift the hips up off of the floor on the inhaling breath. Lift the head and look toward the nose—nasa drishti. Keep the hips and knees lifted up off of the floor. Stay here in Kukkutasana for five deep breaths.

Place the legs and hips onto the floor. Pull the arms out from between the legs. Either swing back into Chaturanga Dandasana from Padamasana or first straighten the legs and then swing back into Chaturanga Dandasana. Inhale into Urdhva Mukha Shvanasana. Exhale into Adho Mukha Shvanasana. Jump through and sit down.

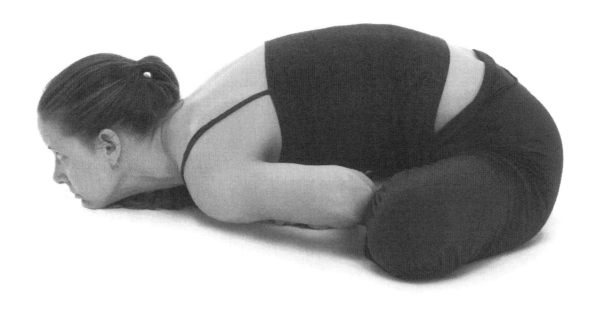

BADDHA KONASANA A

Bend the knees and drop them out to the sides. Press the
outsides of the soles of the feet together and draw the
feet in close to the hips. Hold the feet with the hands and
press the knees down to the floor. Inhale, lift the chest,
and exhale reach the chest forward and down to the floor.
Extend the chin forward and look to the nose—nasa drishti.
The elbows bend and are placed on the legs. Stay here in
Baddha Konasana A for five breaths.

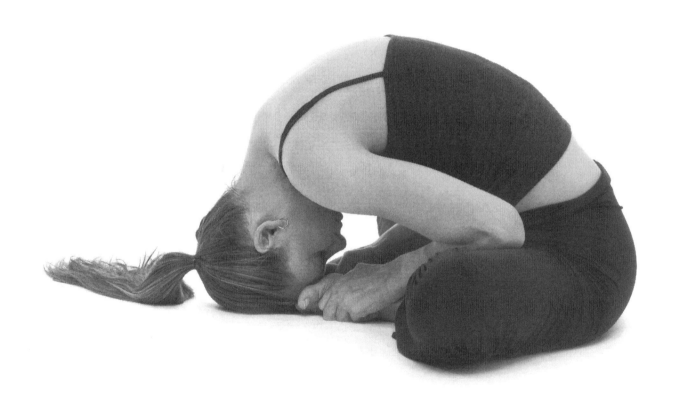

BADDHA KONASANA B

Inhale and lift the head and torso back up to an upright, seated position. Exhale, arch the spine and place the top of the head on the feet or in front of the feet with the forehead touching the toes. Keep the feet close to the hips. Look toward the nose—nasa drishti—and remain here in Baddha Konasana B for five deep breaths.

Inhale and sit back up. Extend the legs out in front of you. Place the palms of the hands on the floor and swing back into Chaturanga Dandansana. Complete the vinyasa and jump back through to sitting.

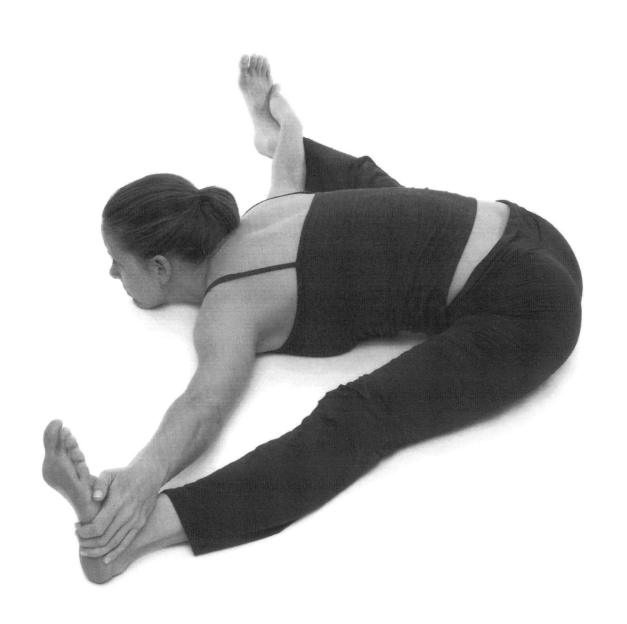

UPAVISHTA KONASANA A

Extend the legs out to the sides. Straighten them and flex
the feet. Bend forward and hold the outsides of the feet
with the hands. Inhale and lift the head and chest until the
arms straighten. Exhale and place the chest on the floor
between the legs, extending the chin forward. Reach the
feet out to the sides, keeping the arms straight. Stay here
for five breaths.

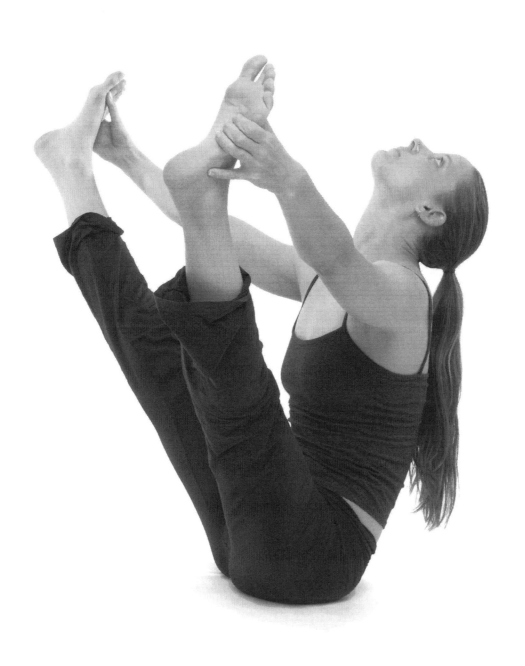

UPAVISHTA KONASANA B

Then, inhale and lift the head, torso and legs up as you balance on the hips. If you can, keep holding the outsides of the feet with the hands throughout the movement. Straighten the arms and legs, lift the chest and drop the head back by reaching the chin up. Look up—urdhva drishti. Remain in this position for five breaths.

Release the feet and place the palms of the hands on the floor on either side of the hips. Exhale, lift the hips and swing back into Chaturanga Dandasana. Complete the vinyasa.

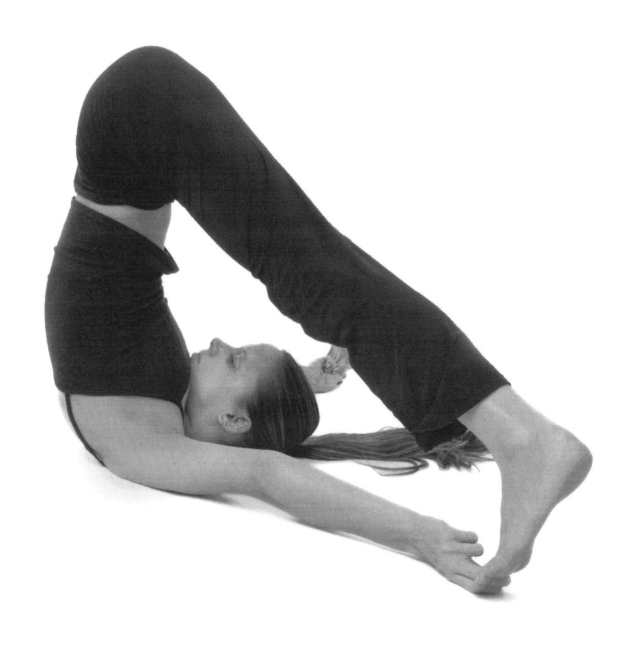

SUPTA KONASANA

Lie down on the back with straight legs and straight arms extended down at your sides. With the palms of the hands facing down, press the arms into the floor and lift the legs and hips as the feet reach up and over the head until the weight is shifted into the shoulders and back of the head. Keep the legs straight and spread them as they extend over the head until the toes touch the floor. Reach the arms, keeping them straight, over the head along the floor. Take hold of the big toes with the first two fingers and thumbs. Lift the hips and look toward the nose—nasa drishti. Stay here for five breaths.

Exhale and drop the hips down to the floor as you rock up to balance on the hips. Keep hold of the toes, the legs spread, the arms and legs straight. Inhale, lift the chest and chin. Straighten the spine. Then, keeping hold of the big toes and the legs straight, flex the feet in order to land on the calves as you drop the legs down to the floor on the exhale. Release the toes and sit up. Press the palms of the hands into the floor and lift the legs and hips to swing back for a vinyasa.

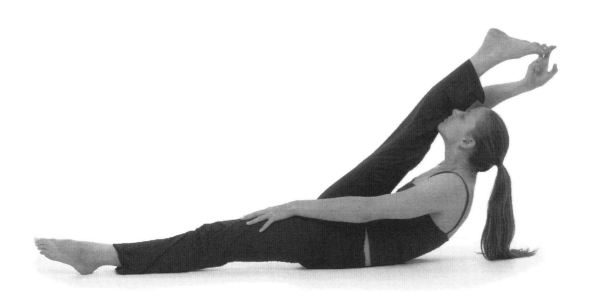

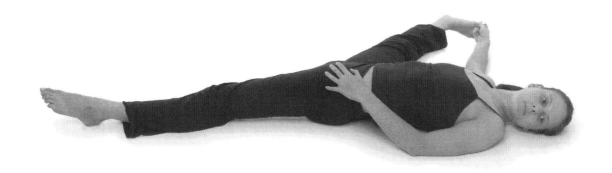

SUPTA PADANGUSTHASANA

Jump through and lie down on the back, with the legs straight and together. Place the palm of the left hand on the top of the left thigh, keeping the left arm straight and pointing the left toes. Keep the right leg straight and lift the right leg all the way up, drawing it down toward the torso. Encircle the right big toe with the first two fingers and thumb of the right hand. Exhaling, lift the torso up to the right leg as you draw the right leg down to the torso with the right arm. Touch the right shin with the chin and look toward the right foot. Look toward the foot —pada drishti. Remain in this position for five breaths. On the exhale place the torso back down on the floor and allow the right arm to straighten. Lower the right leg down to the floor to the right with the arm, keeping them both straight. Rotate the head to the left and look to the nose—nasa drishti. Stay in this asana for five breaths. Inhale and lift the right leg back up. Exhale and touch the chin to the right shin.

Place the torso back down on the floor and release the toe. Lower the right leg back down to the floor next to the left leg.

Switch sides, by placing the palm of the right hand on top of the right thigh and lifting the left leg. Catch the left big toe with the left hand and touch the left shin with the chin on the exhale. Look toward the foot—pada drishti. Remain here for five breaths. Exhale and place the head and torso on the floor, straightening the left arm and lower the left leg down to the floor on the left. Rotate the head to the right and look toward the nose—nasa drishti. Stay in this position for five breaths. On the inhale lift the left leg back up to the previous position and touch the chin to the left shin on the exhale. Place the torso back down on the floor and release the toe. Lower the left leg down to the floor next to the right leg.

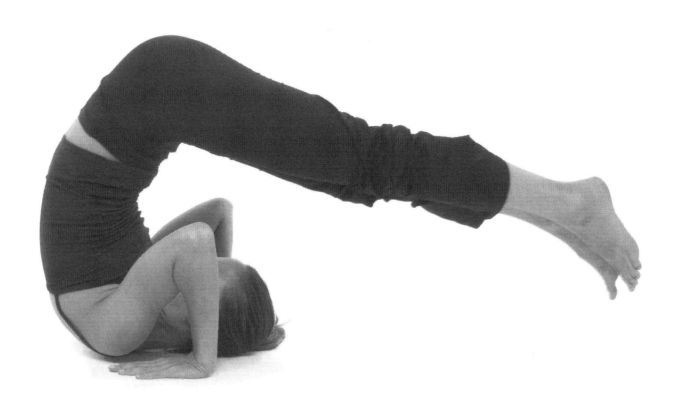

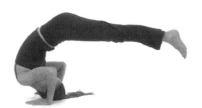

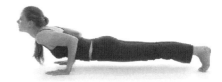

CHAKRASANA

Place the arms, with the palms of the hands facing down, on the floor to either side of the torso. On the exhale, lift the legs and swing them up and over head by pressing into the arms. Allow the torso the curl up off of the floor. When only the back of the head and shoulders contact the floor, place the palms of the hands on the floor to either side of the head, with the elbows bent and lifted and the fingers pointing toward the shoulders. Continue reaching the legs back over and away from the head and look toward the nose. As you press the hands into the floor, lift the shoulders and head off of the floor into Chaturanga Dandaasana as the feet flex and the toes make contact with the floor. Inhale into Urdhva Mukha Shvanasana. Exhale into Adho Mukha Shvanasana. Jump back through the arms.

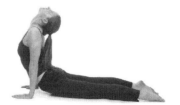
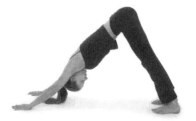

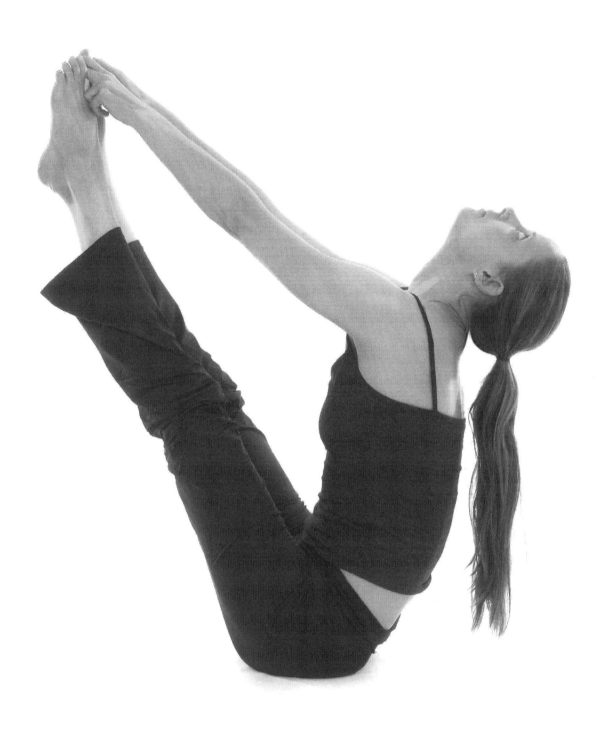

UBHAYA PADANGUSTHASANA

Lie down on the back with the legs straight and together. Keeping the legs straight, lift them up off of the floor and reach them over the head on the exhale. Allow the hips and back to lift up off of the floor. Touch the toes to the floor and reach the arms up over the head. Encircle the big toes with the first two fingers and thumbs. Inhale, drop the hips back down to the floor and rock up to a seated position, keeping the arms and legs straight throughout the movement. Balance on the hips and straighten the spine by lifting the chest. Drop the head back by lifting the chin, and look up—urdhva drishti. Stay in Ubhaya Padangusthasana for five breaths. Place the palms of the hands on the floor on either side of the hips. Press into the palms of the hands and bend the legs. Lift the hips up off of the floor. Swing the hips and legs back through the arms into Chaturanga Dandasana. Inhale into Urdhva Mukha Shvanasana. Exhale into Adho Mukha Shvanasana.

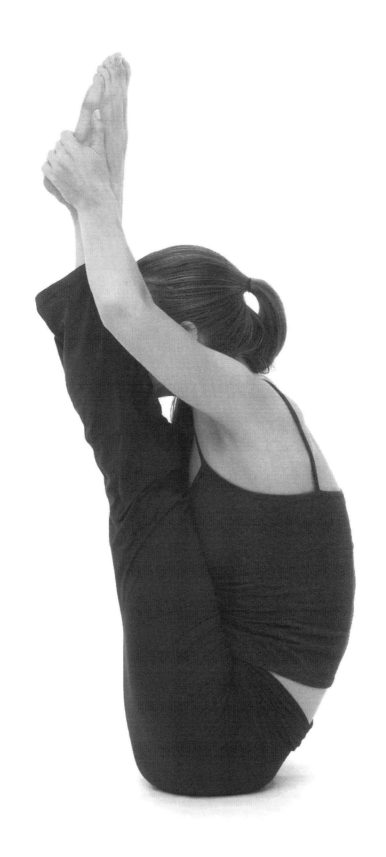

URDHVA MUKHA PASCHIMOTTANASANA

Jump through the arms and lie down on the back. Keeping the legs straight, lifting them up off of the floor. Reach them over the head on the exhale and allow the hips and back to lift up off of the floor. Touch the toes to the floor and reach the arms up over the head. Hold the outsides of the feet. Inhale and drop the hips down to the floor and rock up to an upright position, keeping hold of the outsides of the feet and the arms and legs straight. Balance on the hips. Use the arms to pull the chest and legs together by bending the elbows. Lift the chin and look toward the feet—pada drishti. Stay here for five breaths. Then, release the feet and place the palms of the hands on the floor to either side of the hips. Bend the knees and press into the palms of the hands to lift the hips. Swing the legs and hips back through the arms into Chaturanga Dandasana without touching the floor with the feet. Inhale into Urdhva Mukha Shvanasana. Exhale into Adho Mukha Shavanasana.

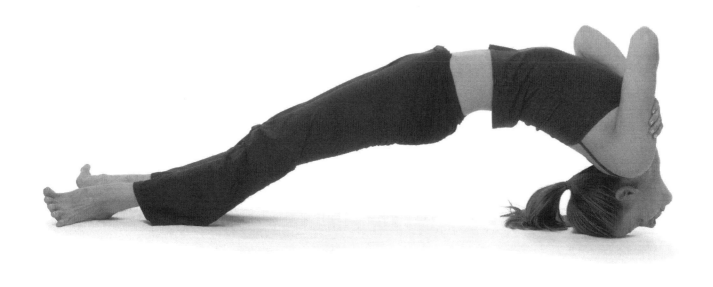

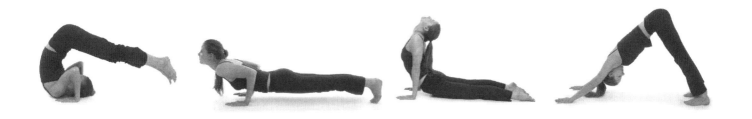

SETU BANDHASANA

Jump through the arms and lie down on the back, with the legs straight and together. Bend the knees slightly and rotate the legs externally until the sides of the feet contact the floor. Keep the heels of the feet together. Lift the chest by pressing the elbows into the floor. Drop the head back and place the top of the head on the floor. Press down and away with the feet to lift the hips and straighten the legs. Allow the chest to lift up above the head and the weight of the body to drop down through the top of the head. Straighten the legs completely until the knees touch, keeping the heels of the feet together. Lift the arms and cross them over the chest by placing the hands on the shoulders. Keep the elbows in contact with the chest. Look to the nose and stay in Setu Bandhasana for five deep breaths. Then, place the hips back down on the floor. Press the elbows into the floor to support the neck as you lift the chest and head off of the floor. Draw the chin in toward the chest and roll the spine down onto the floor. Straighten the legs, and place the arms down alongside the body with the palms of the hands on the floor in preparation for Chakrasana. Exhale into Chaturanga Dandasana by moving through Chakrasana. Inhale into Urdhva Mukha Shvanasana. Exhale into Adho Mukha Shvanasana.

Setu Bandhasana is the last Primary Series Asana. When practicing the Primary Series continue with the finishing asanas, starting with Urdhva Dhanurasana.

The intermediate series is referred to as Nadi Shodhana. Nadi is translated as little river. The nadies are a network of energy channels which underlie the physical body. Shodhana means to purify, cleanse or eliminate obstructions. The intermediate series is designed to strengthen and purify the nervous system.

It is of the utmost importance to practice the primary series for several years until all of the asanas and vinyasas of this series are deeply integrated into the body before commencing the practice of the intermediate series. The asanas of the primary series lengthen the spine, strengthen the abdominal muscles and open the hips, knees and ankles. This prepares the body for practicing the intermediate series safely and effectively.

Sthira Sukham Asanam.
Yoga postures are to be steady and pleasurable.
Yoga Sutras – Chapter 2, Verse 46

INTERMEDIATE SERIES

The practice of the postures of the intermediate series begins when all the asanas of the primary series are comfortable and the breath is smooth throughout the practice.

The postures of the intermediate series are introduced one asana at a time to the primary series after completing Setubandhasana and prior to practicing Urdhva Dhanurasana. When all of the asanas up to Tittibhasana have been added to the Primary Series, the asanas of the primary series from Parshvottanasana to Setu Bandhasana are dropped. The remaining asanas of the intermediate series are then added without the primary series, which is practiced independently once a week, traditionally on Fridays.

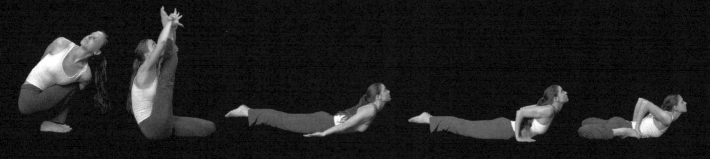

PASHASANA   KROUNCHASANA   A   B   BHEKASANA

SHALABHASANA

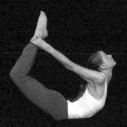 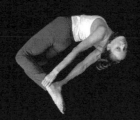 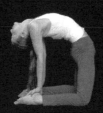 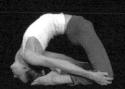

DHANURASANA   PARSHVA   USTRASANA   LAGHUVAJRASANA
                    DHANURASANA

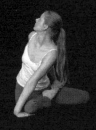 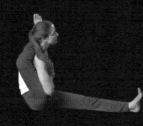 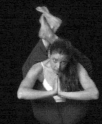 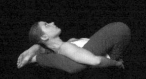

BHARADHVA-   A   B   DWI PADA   YOGA NIDRASANA
JASANA   EKA PADA SHIRSHASANA   SHIRSHASANA

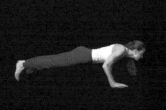 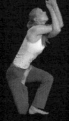 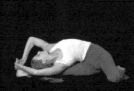 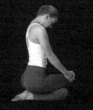 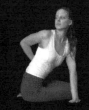

NAKRASANA   VATAYANASANA   PARIGASANA   A   B   SUPTA URDHVA
                                                      GOMUKHASANA   VAJRASANA

INTERMEDIATE SERIES

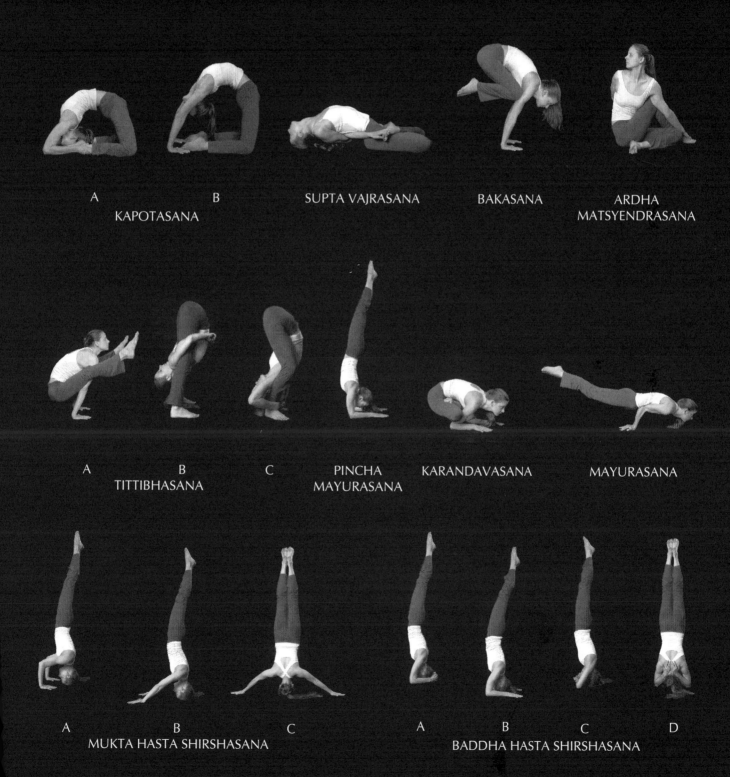

A   B   SUPTA VAJRASANA   BAKASANA   ARDHA
KAPOTASANA   MATSYENDRASANA

A   B   C   PINCHA   KARANDAVASANA   MAYURASANA
TITTIBHASANA   MAYURASANA

A   B   C   A   B   C   D
MUKTA HASTA SHIRSHASANA   BADDHA HASTA SHIRSHASANA

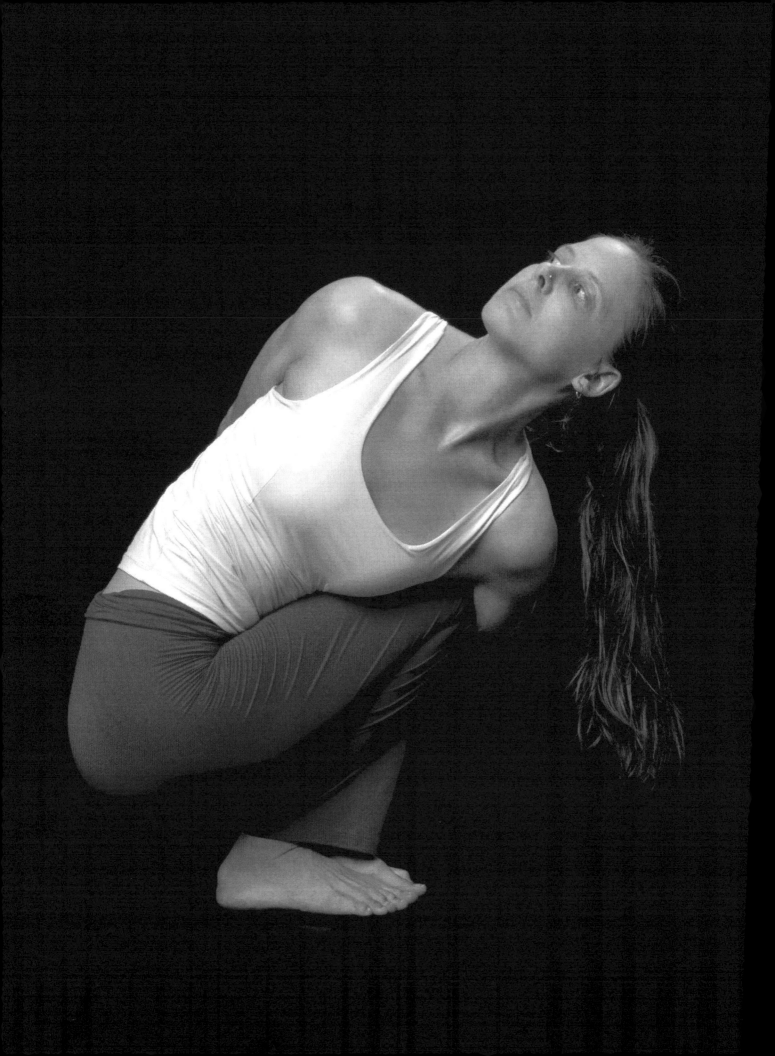

PASHASANA

When this asana is first practiced it is added after Setubandhasana. From Adho Mukha Shvanasana, jump forward between the hands on an exhale and land on the feet in a squatted position with the feet together. Once the primary series asanas are dropped, enter Pashasana after completing Parshvottanasana by practicing Surya Namaskara A up to Adho Mukha Shvanasana and then jump forward between the hands into a squatted position with the feet together on an exhale.

Lift the right arm on an inhale. Exhale, twist to the left and draw the right elbow down to the outside of the left thigh, allowing the elbow to bend. Keep the heel on the floor. Then, rotate the right arm internally and wrap the arm around the legs. Reach back and clasp the left wrist with the right hand. Twist the head to the left and set the gaze—parshva drishti. Remain here for five deep breaths. Inhale, release the clasp of the right hand on the left wrist and rotate forward. Then, enter Pashasana on the right side by lifting the left arm and twisting to the left. Wrap the left arm around the legs, reach the right arm back and clasp the right wrist with the left hand. Rotate the head to the right and set the gaze—parshva drishti. Stay here for five breaths.

Inhale, release the arms and rotate forward. Place the palms of the hands on the floor next to the feet. Jump back into Chaturanga Dandasana on the exhale. Inhale, Urdhva Mukha Shvanasana. Exhale, Adho Mukha Shvanasana.

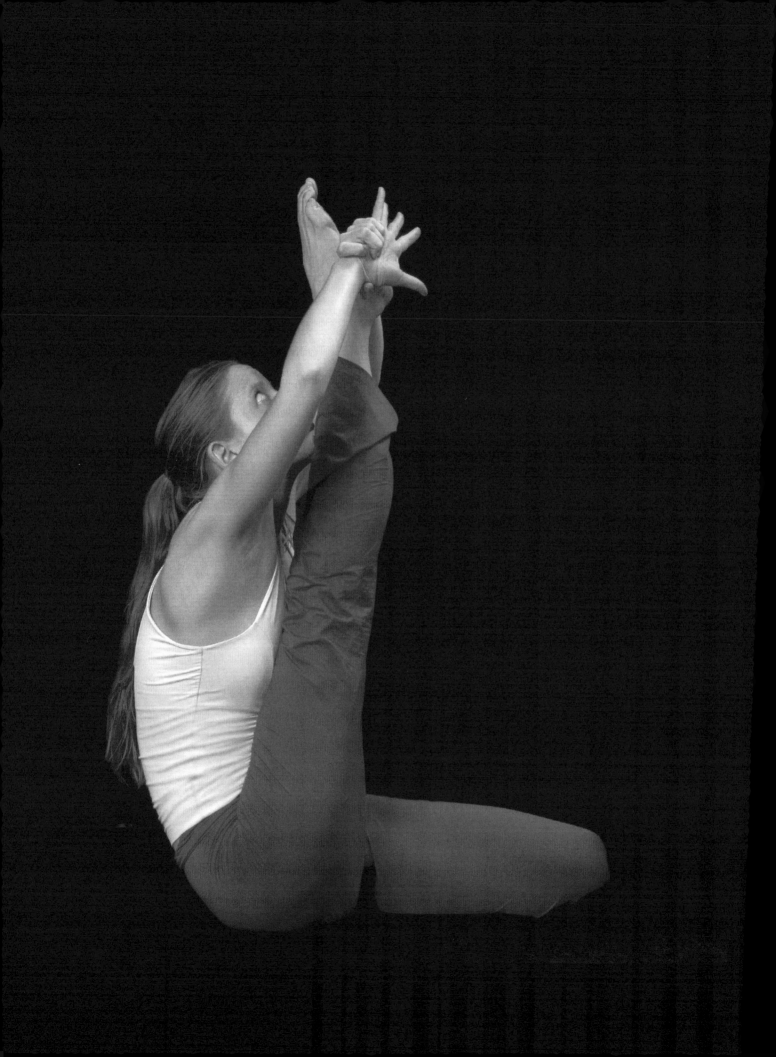

KROUNCHASANA

Enter Krounchasana by jumping through the arms with the left leg bent and the toes pointing back. The knee extends forward next to the right leg, which remains straight. When the hips land on the floor between the hands, the left knee is bent with the top of the left foot against the floor, and the right leg is straight and raised forty-five degrees off of the floor. Lift the arms and clasp the left wrist with the right hand around the right foot. Inhale, lift the chest to straighten the spine, tilt the head back and straighten the arms. Exhale and using the arms raise the right leg until it is perpendicular to the floor. Point the right toes, place the chest and chin on the right leg and look up to the right foot –pada drishti. Stay in the asana for five breaths.

Inhale, straighten the arms and tilt the head back. Exhale, place the palms of the hands on the floor on either side of the hips and swing back into Chaturanga Dandasana. Inhale into Urdhva Mukha Shvanasana. Exhale, pushing up to Adho Mukha Shvanasana.

Jump through for the left side, keeping the right leg bent with the knee extended forward next to the left leg, which is kept straight. Raise the left leg and clasp the right wrist with the left hand around the left leg. Inhale, lift the chest to straighten the spine and tilt the head back allowing the arms to straighten. Exhale, raise the left leg by bending the arms and place the chest and chin on the left leg. Point the toes on the left foot and look up toward it—pada drishti. Stay in Pashasana on the left side for five deep breaths. Inhale, straighten the arms, lift the chest and tilt the head back. Exhale, place the palms of the hands on the floor next to the hips and swing back into Chaturanga Dandanasana. Inhale, Urdhva Mukha Shvanasana. Exhale, Adho Mukha Shvanasana.

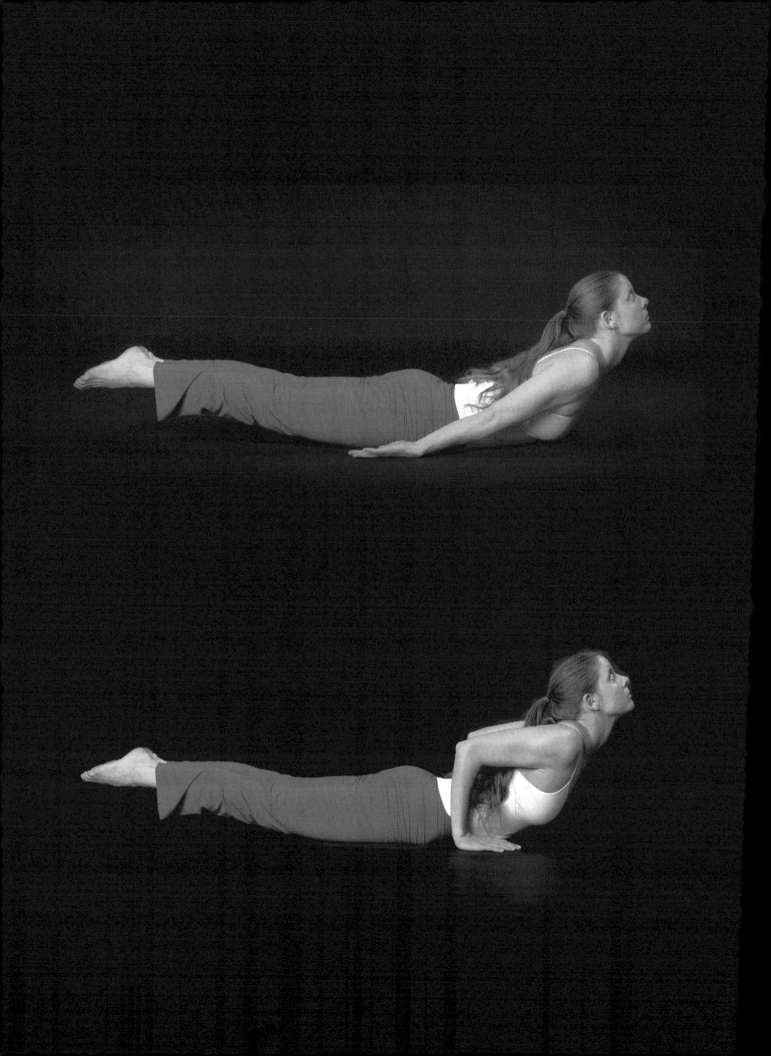

SHALABHASANA A & B

A: Return to Chaturanga Dandasana on the exhale, lowering the pelvis and abdomen onto the floor. Inhale, raise the legs and draw them together. pointing the toes. Keep the legs straight and the chest and head lifted. Extend the arms back on either side of the torso with the palms of the hands facing up. Keeping the arms straight, press the backs of the hands into the floor gently. Lift the chin and look to the nose–nasa drishti. Stay here for five smooth breaths.

B: Keep the legs lifted. Bend the elbows and place the palms of the hands on the floor on either side of the waist so that the forearms are perpendicular to the floor. Press the hands into the floor. Draw the elbows toward each other so that the upper arms are parallel. Lift the chest higher. Lift the chin and look to the nose—nasa drishti. Stay here for five deep breaths.

Place the tops of the feet on the floor, straighten the arms and pull the chest forward and up into Urdhva Mukha Shvanasana. Exhale, Adho Mukha Shvanasana.

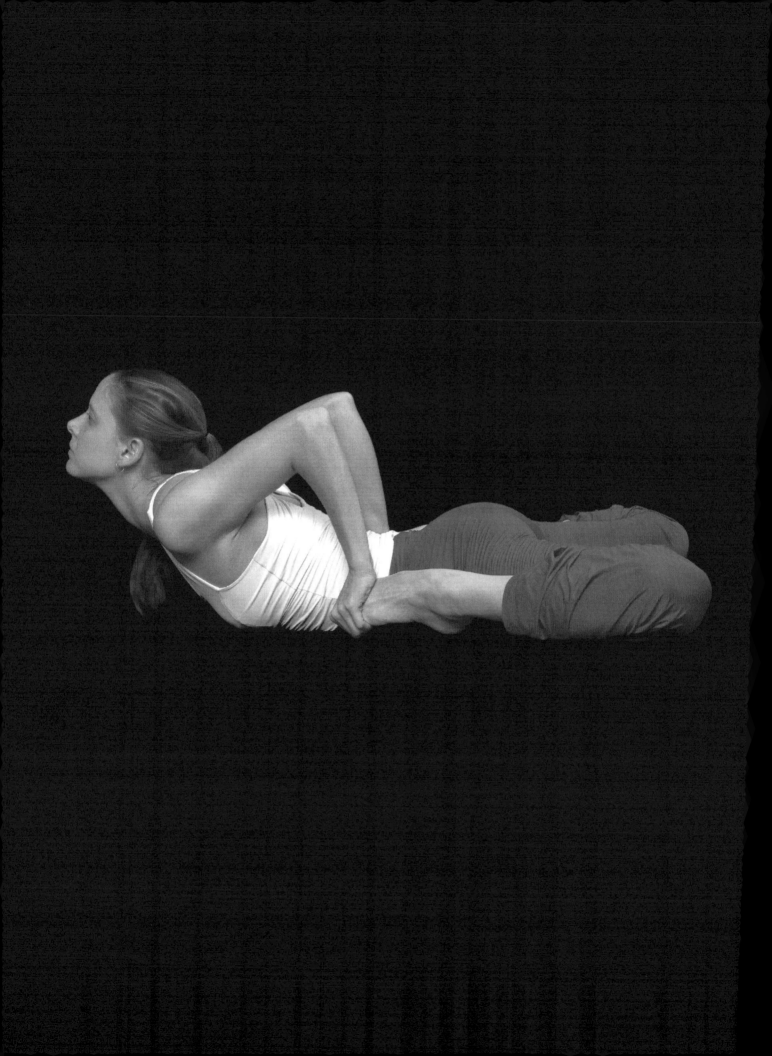

BHEKASANA

Exhaling, lower into Chaturanga Dandasana. Place the pelvis
and abdomen on the floor. Bend the knees, and reach the arms
back, rotating them externally until the palms of the hands
face out and the thumbs point up. Take hold of the insides of
the feet. Bend and lift the elbows, rotating the arms internally.
Rotate the hands so that the palms of the hands press the tops
of the feet down until the heels touch the floor. Lift the chest
and chin, and look toward the nose—nasa drishti. Remain in the
asana for five breaths.

Place the palms of the hands on the floor on either side of the
waist, straighten the legs and press the tops of the feet into
the floor. Straighten the arms, and reach the chest forward
and up into Urdhva Mukha Shvanasana. Exhale, Adho Mukha
Shvanasana.

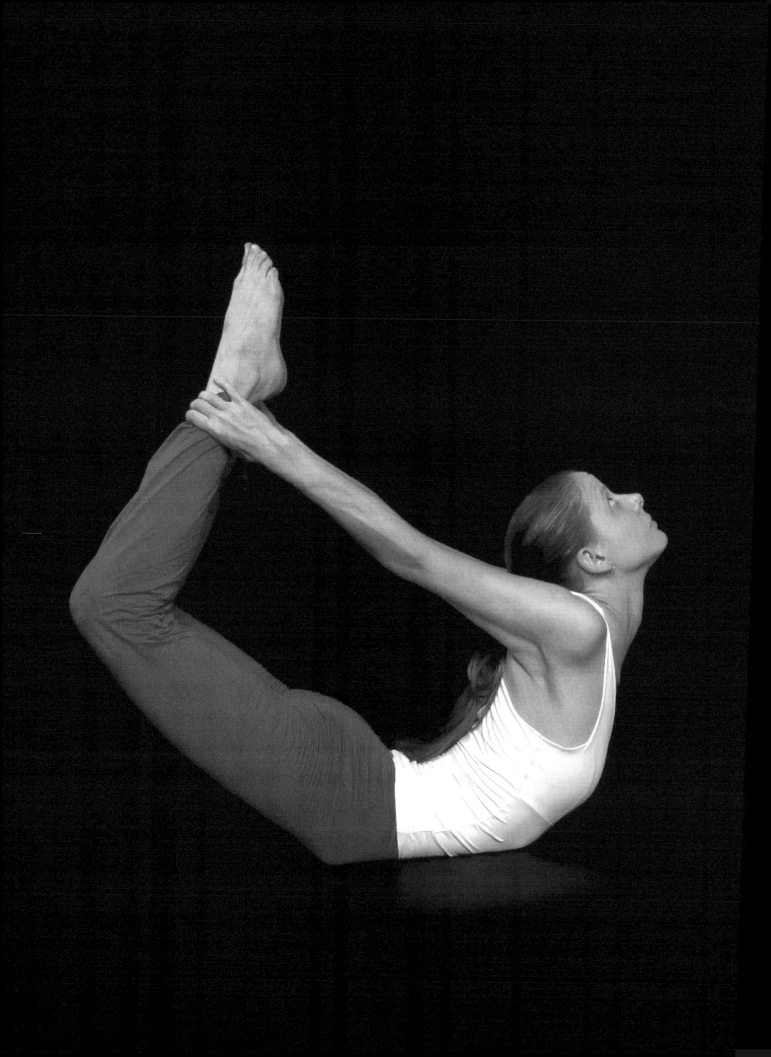

DHANURASANA

Exhale, lowering into Chaturanga Dandasana. Place the pelvis and abdomen on the floor. Bend the knees and reach the arms back, rotating the forearm externally until the palms of the hands face each other and the thumbs point down. Take hold of the outsides of the lower legs, just below the ankles. Point the toes, and press the feet together. Draw the knees toward each other until they're about hip width apart. Lift the feet up toward the sky by pressing the lower legs into the hands, keeping the arms straight. Allow the thighs to lift up off of the floor. Arch the spine, and lift the chest. Tilt the head back and look to the forehead—ajna drishti. Stay here for five deep breaths.

Lower the thighs to the floor, and release the hands, placing the palms on the floor at either side of the waist. Extend the legs, and press the tops of the feet into the floor. Straighten the arms and reach the chest forward and up into Urdhva Mukha Shvanasana. Exhale, Adho Mukha Shvanasana.

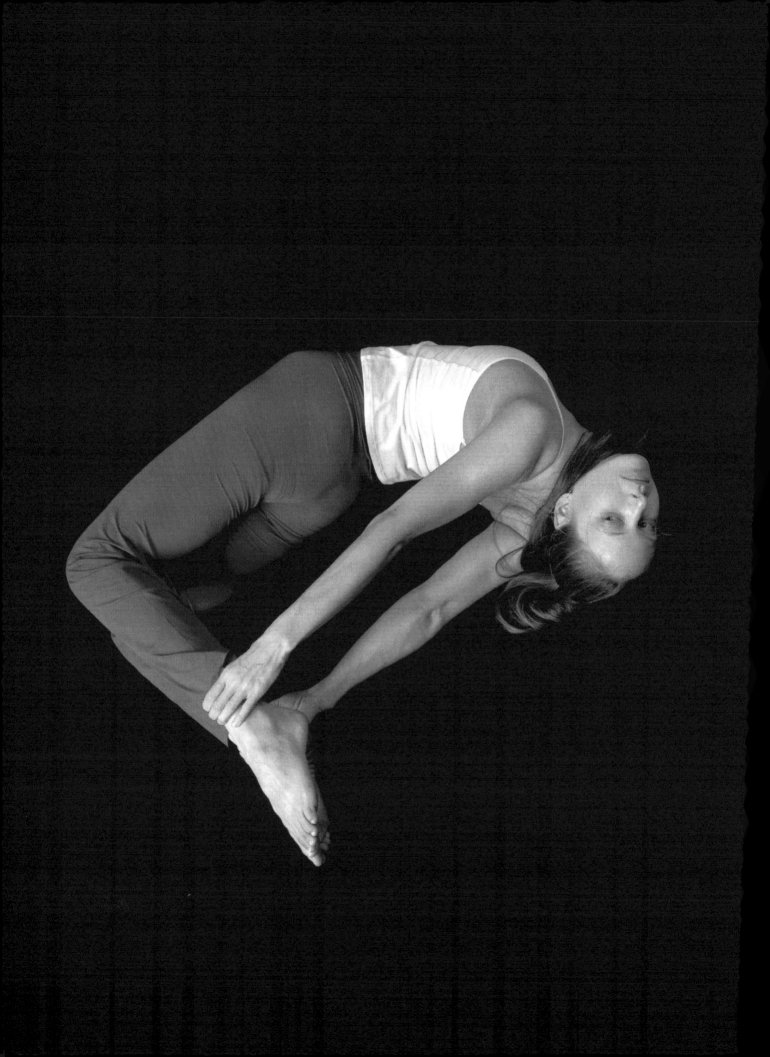

PARSHVA DHANURASANA

Exhale, lowering into Chaturanga Dandasana. Place the pelvis and abdomen on the floor. Take hold of the ankles and inhale into Dhanurasana. Exhale, rock to the right, retaining a deep arch in the spine and keeping the feet in contact with each other and lower the body down to the floor, to the right. Draw the feet away from the shoulders and look towards the feet—parshva drishti. Remain in Parshva Dhanurasana for five deep breaths. Inhale, raise the body back up into Dhanurasana, while keeping the feet in contact with each other. Exhale, rock to the left and lower the body down to the floor, to the left. Retain the arch in the spine and keep the feet in contact with each other. Lift the chin away from the sternum and look towards the feet— parshva drishti. Remain in Parshva Dhanurasana for five breaths. Inhale, raise the body back up into Dhanurasana, while keeping the feet in contact with each other. Tilt the head back and look to the forehead—ajna drishti. Stay here for five deep breaths.

Lower the thighs to the floor, and release the hands, placing the palms on the floor at either side of the waist. Extend the legs, and press the tops of the feet into the floor. Straighten the arms and reach the chest forward and up into Urdhva Mukha Shvanasana. Exhale, Adho Mukha Shvanasana.

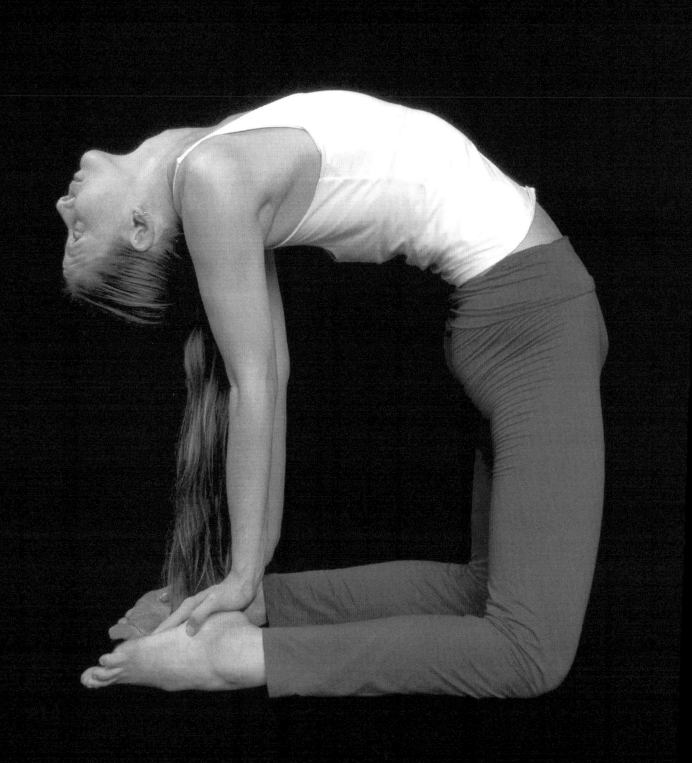

USTRASANA

Exhale, jump forward between the hands and bend the knees, landing on the lower legs with the knees hips width apart and toes pointing back. Inhale and lift the hips above the knees, raising the torso to an upright position. Place the hands on the hips, and lift the chest. Lift the chin, and drop the head back. Exhale, rotate the arms externally and place the palms on the soles of the feet with the fingers pointing back. Look to the forehead—ajna drishti. Remain here for five deep breaths. On the inhale, shift the weight of the hips forward. Raise the chest, keeping the head dropped back until the torso reaches an upright position. Place the palms of the hands together in front of the chest, and lift the head up. Lower the chin. Place the palms of the hands on either side of the knees. Jump back into Chaturanga Dandasana. Inhale, Urdhva Mukha Shvanasana. Exhale, Adho Mukha Shvanasana.

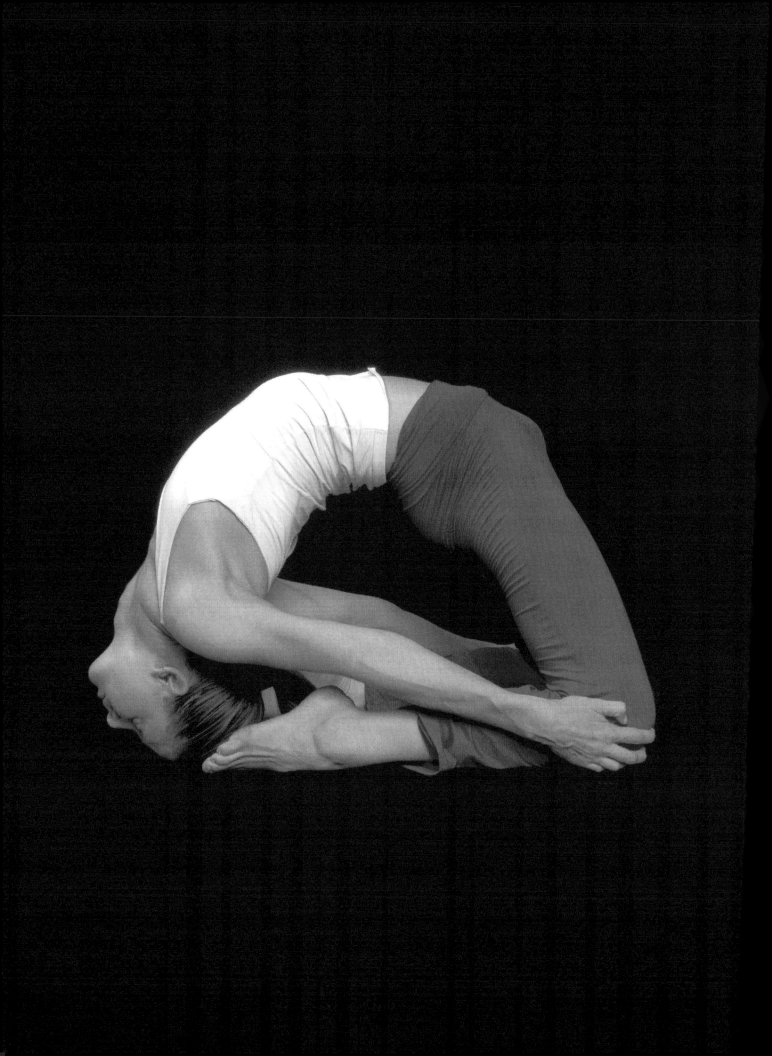

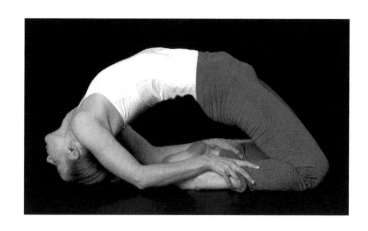

LAGHUVAJRASANA

Exhale and jump forward between the hands, coming onto the knees. Inhale, raise up on the knees and lift the chest, placing the hands on the hips. Lift the chin and tilt the head back. Shift the weight of the hips forward and arch the spine. Drop the arms and reach back towards the knees. On the exhale, lower the top of the head down to the floor using the strength of the legs. Take hold of the knees or the upper calf, just below the knees. Look up to the forehead—ajna drishti. Remain in this asana for five breaths.

Inhale, press the lower legs and tops of the feet into the floor to pull the hips above the knees and align the chest above the hips, keeping the head tilted back. Then, lift the head by lowering the chin as you raise the arms and bring the palms of the hands together in front of the chest.

Place the hands on the floor on either side of the knees. Jump back into Chaturanga Dandasana. Inhale, Urdhva Mukha Shvanasana. Exhale, Adho Mukha Shvanasana.

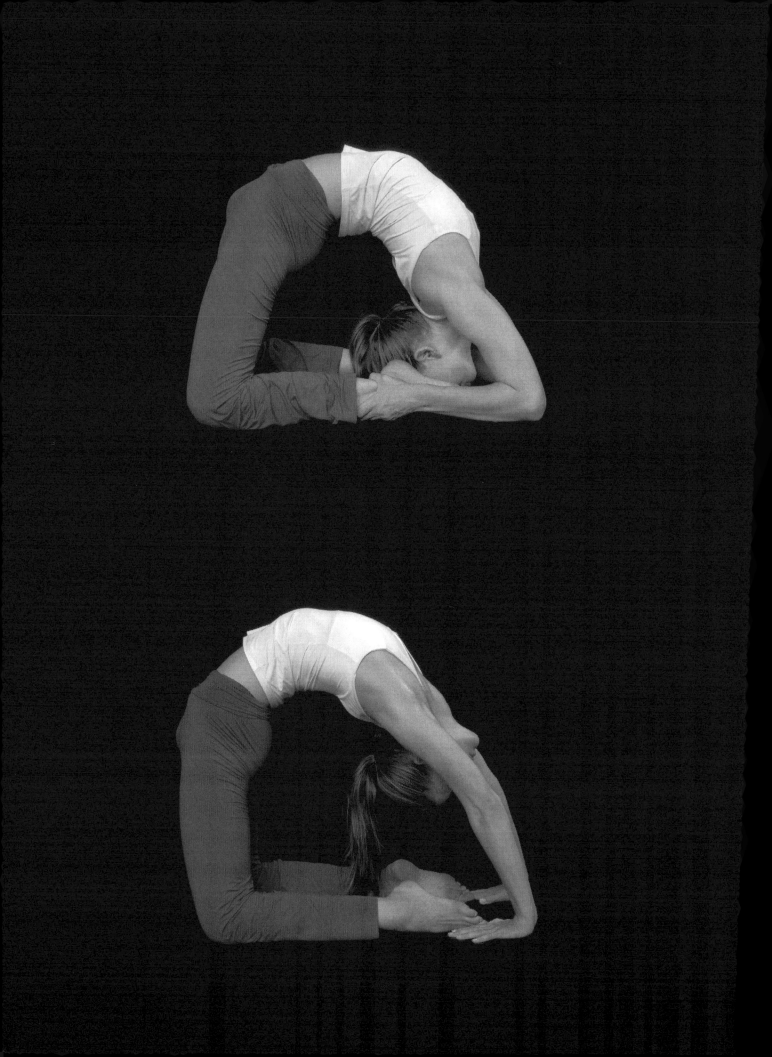

KAPOTASANA A & B

Exhale, jump forward onto the knees. Inhale, stand up on the knees and lift the chest, placing the hands on the hips. Bring the palms of the hands together in front of the chest, lift the chin, drop the head back and arch the spine. Exhale, and lower the head down toward the floor while raising the arms above the head and reaching toward the feet. Keep the thighs parallel to each other. Take hold of the heels or the ankles. Drop the elbows and the forehead to the floor, keeping the arms parallel to each other. Look up to the forehead–ajna drishti. Stay here for five breaths. Then, place the palms of the hands on the floor on either side of the toes. Inhale and straighten the arms. Remain in this position for five deep breaths.

Inhale, raise the torso back up, lifting the head last, and bring the palms of the hands together in front of the chest. Place the palms of the hands on the floor on either side of the knees. Exhale, hop back into Chaturanga Dandasana. Inhale, Urdhva Mukha Shvanasana. Exhale, Adho Mukha Shvanasana.

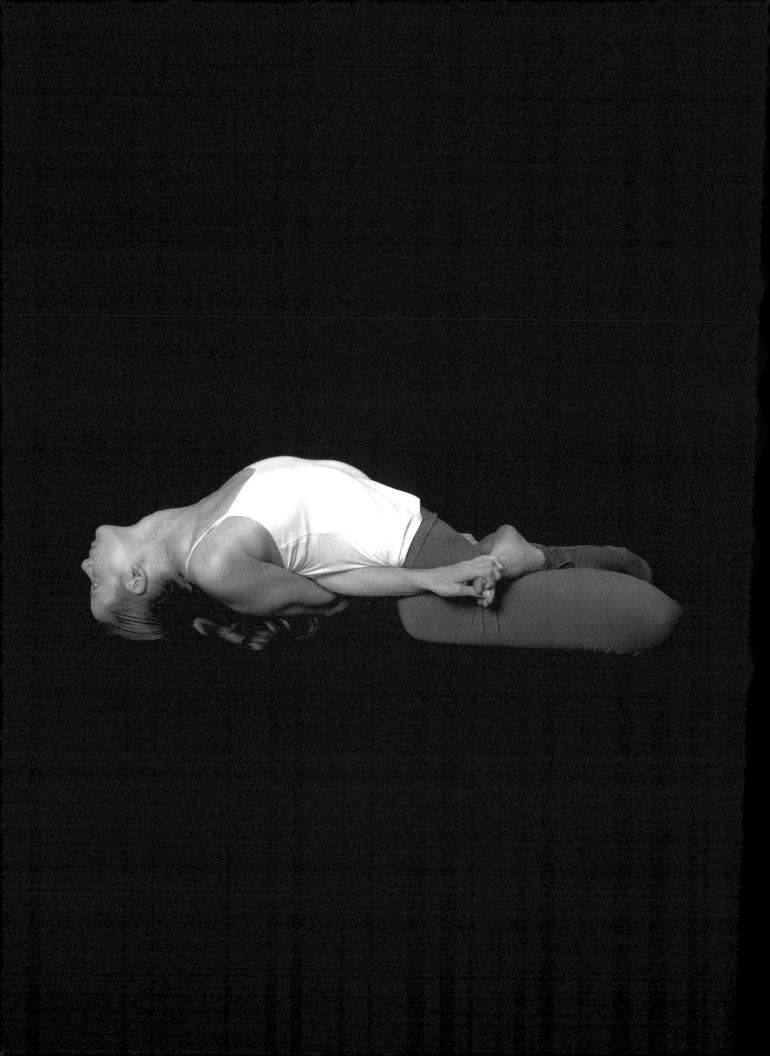

SUPTA VAJRASANA

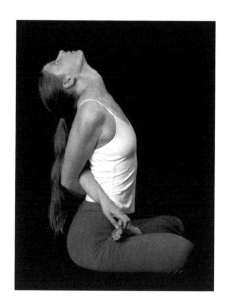

Jump through the arms and sit down. Enter Padmasana by placing the right foot in the crease of the left hip and then the left foot in the crease of the right hip. Reach the left arm behind the back and encircle the left big toe with the first two fingers of the left hand, completing the circle with the thumb. Reach the right arm behind the back and encircle the right big toe with the first two fingers of the right hand, completing the circle with the thumb.

Lift the chest and chin, and drop the head back. The knees need to be secured on the floor, either by another person or an object. On the exhale, lower the torso back and down until the top of the head touches the floor. Look up to the forehead—ajna drishti. Remain in the asana for five deep breaths. Inhale and raise the torso back up to seated, keeping the head tilted back. Exhale back down. Inhale up. Exhale down. Inhale up. Exhale back down, and again stay in the asana for five breaths. Then inhale back up and lift the head as you lower the chin.

Release the arms. Place the palms of the hands on the floor on either side of the hips. Swing back into Chaturanga Dandasana. Inhale, Urdhva Mukha Shvanasana. Exhale, Adho Mukha Shvanasana.

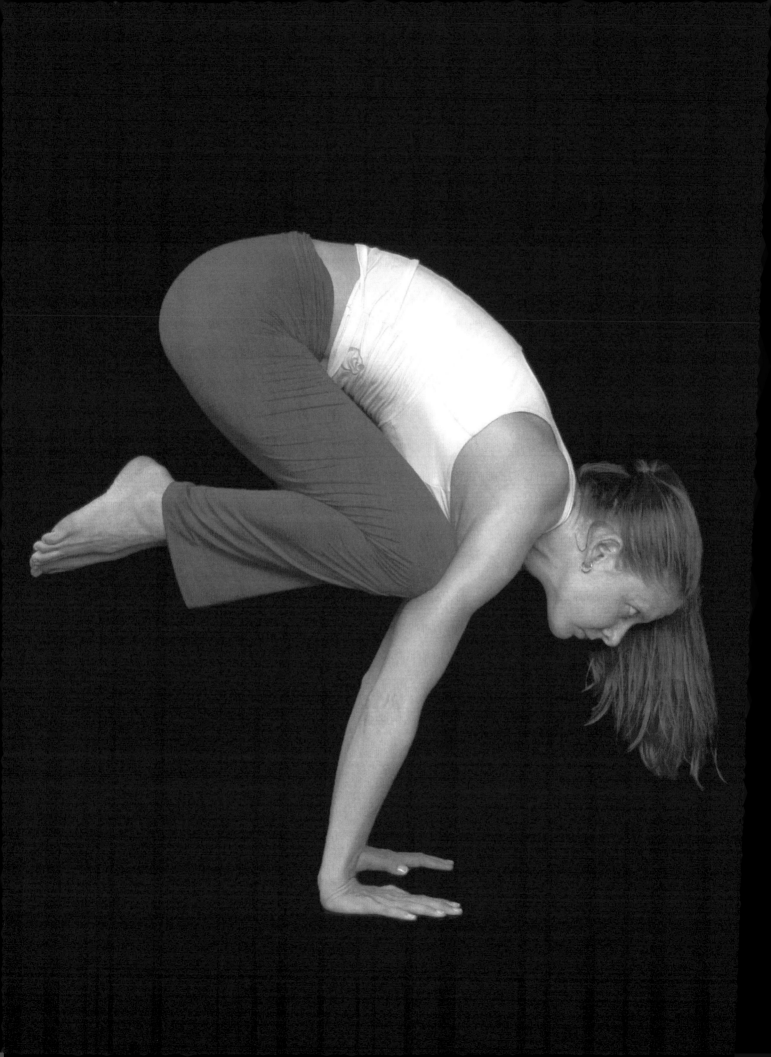

BAKASANA A & B

Exhale, jump forward between the hands into a squatting position with the feet together and the knees apart. Drop the torso down between the thighs. Place the palms of the hands on the floor just aside the feet with the upper arms underneath the shins. Inhale, lift the hips and legs by straightening the arms. Keep the feet in contact and point the toes back. Bend the knees and lift the feet. Lift the head and look towards the tip of the nose—nasa drishti. Remain in Bakasana for five breaths.

Exhale, jump back into Chaturanga Dandasana. Inhale Urdhva Mukha Shvanasana. Exhale Adho Mukha Shvanasana.

Then lift the head, look forward and jump into Bakasana without touching the feet to the floor on the exhale. Inhale, lift the head and feet, and point the toes. Look to the nose—nasa drishti. Stay in Bakasana for five breaths. Exhale, jump back into Chaturanga Dandasana. Inhale Urdhva Mukha Shvasana. Exhale Adho Mukha Shvanasana.

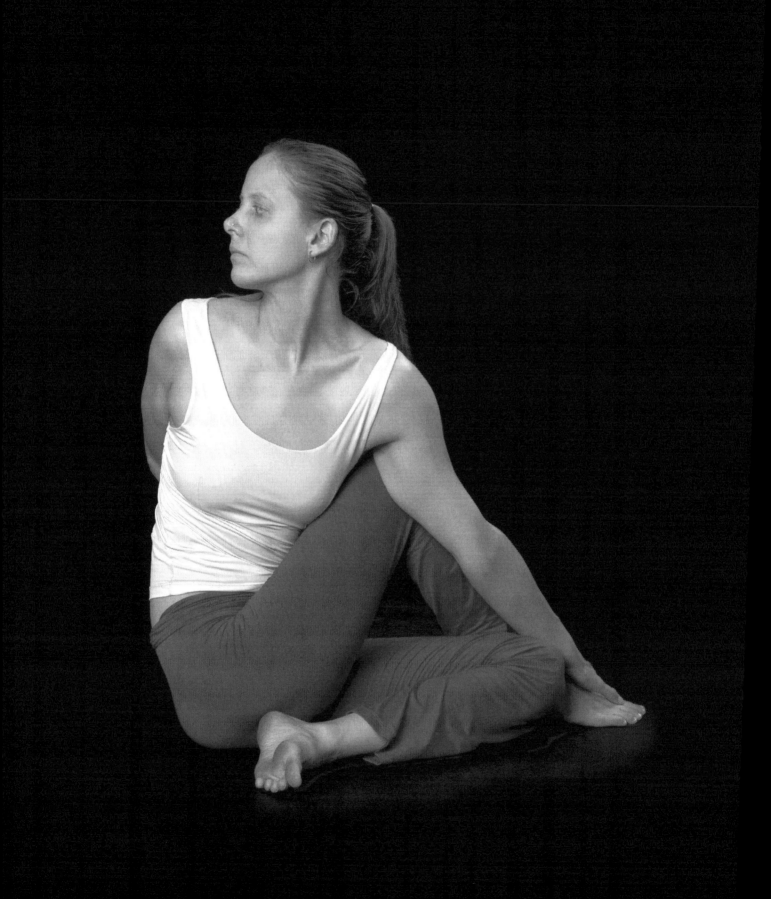

ARDHA MATSYENDRASANA

Jump through and sit down. Bend the knees, crossing the right leg over the left. Place the left foot on the floor to the right of the right hip and drop the left knee to the floor. Place the sole of the right foot to the left of the left knee, keeping the right knee upright. Exhale, twist to the right and place the left elbow to the side of the right leg. Straighten the left arm and take hold of the inside of the right foot with the left hand. Reach the right arm behind you and take hold of the left hip with the right hand. Rotate the head to the left and look to the left—parshva drishti. Remain in this asana for five deep breaths.

Release the arms and rotate the torso forward. Place the palms of the hands on the floor on either side of the hips. Swing back into Chaturanga Dandasana. Inhale, Urdhva Mukha Shvanasana.

Exhale, Adho Mukha Shvanasana. Jump through and sit down.

Bend the knees, placing the right foot to the left of the left hip and the sole of the left foot to the right of the left knee. Place the palm of the left hand on the floor behind you, rotate to the left and place the right elbow to the left of the left knee. Straighten the right arm and take hold of the inside of the left foot. Reach the left arm behind you and take hold of the right hip. Rotate the head to the left and focus the gaze—parshva drishti. Remain in this asana for five deep breaths.

Inhale, release the arms and rotate the spine forward. Place the palms of the hands on the floor next to the hips. Swing back into Chaturanga Dandasana. Inhale, Urdhva Mukha Shvanasana. Exhale, Adho Mukha Shvanasana.

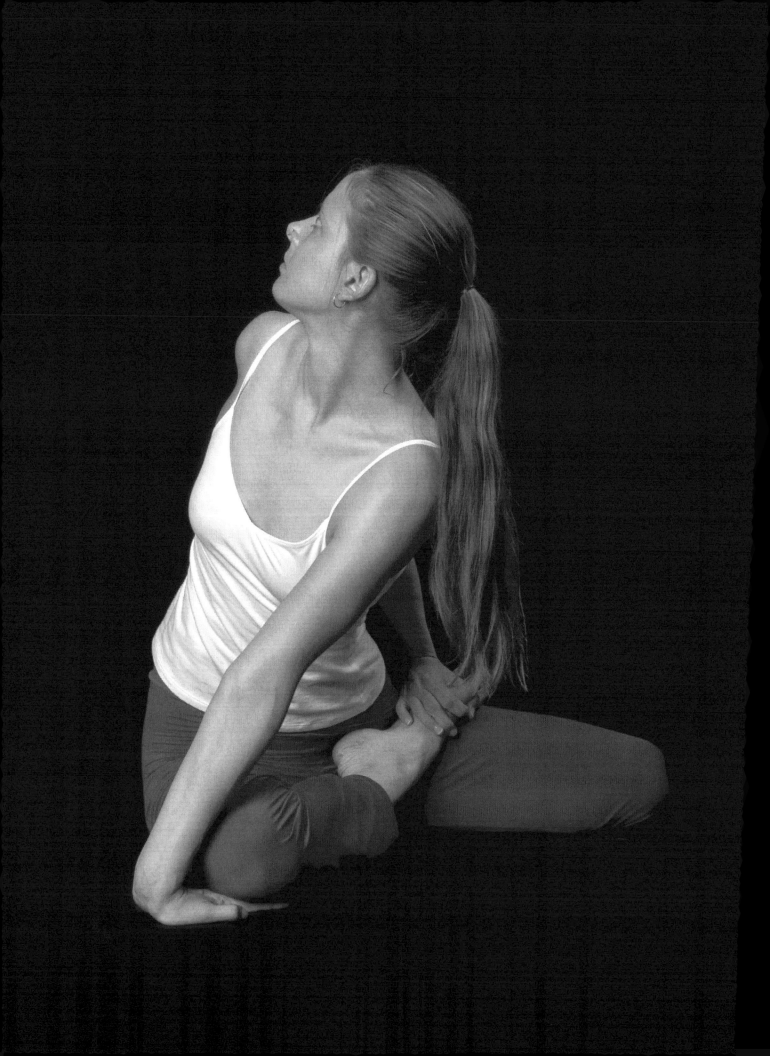

BHARADHVAJASANA

Jump through and sit down. Bend the left leg, place the top of the left foot on the floor to the left of the left hip and drop the left knee to the floor. Bend the right leg and place the top of the right foot on the top of the left thigh. Drop the right knee to the floor ninety degrees to the right. Twist to the right. Reach the right arm behind the back and take hold of the right big toe with the first two fingers of the right hand and encircle the toe with the thumb. Place the palm of the left hand underneath the right knee. Rotate the head to the right and look to the right—parshva drishti. Stay in this asana for five deep breaths.

Release the arms and rotate the torso forward. Jump back into Chaturanga Dandasana. Inhale into Urdhva Mukha Shvanasana. Exhale, Adho Mukha Shvanasana.

Jump through and sit down. Bend the right leg, place the top of the right foot on the floor to the right of the right hip and drop the right knee to the floor. Bend the left leg and place the top of the left foot on the top of the right thigh. Drop the left knee to the floor ninety degrees to the left. Twist to the left. Reach the left arm behind the back and take hold of the left big toe with the first two fingers of the left hand and encircle the toe with the thumb. Place the palm of the right hand underneath the right knee. Rotate the head to the left and look to the right—parshva drishti. Stay in the asana for five deep breaths.

Release the arms and untwist the spine. Jump back into Chaturanga Dandasana. Inhale, Urdhva Mukha Shvanasana. Exhale, Adho Mukha Shvanasana.

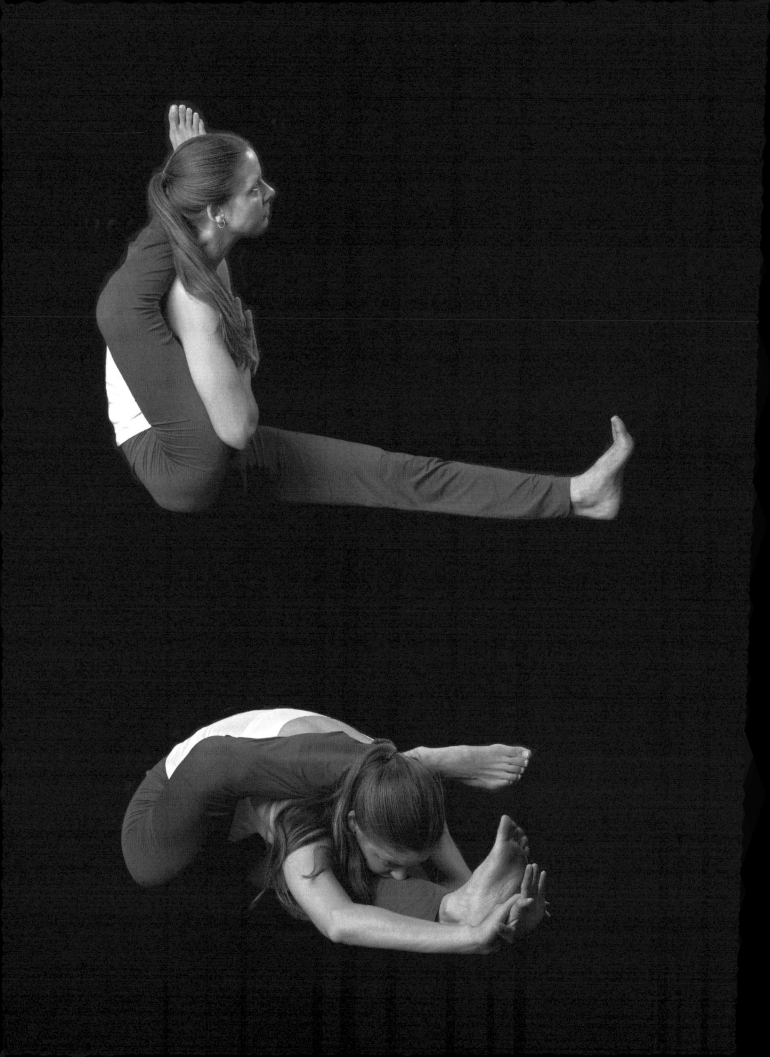

EKA PADA SHIRSHASANA

Jump forward with the left leg keeping it straight between the arms as you move the right leg to the right of the right arm. Take hold of the right foot with the left hand and place the lower right leg behind the head. Straighten the left leg and flex the left foot. Bring the palms of the hand together in front of the chest. Look towards the left foot—pada drishti. Remain here for five deep breaths. Then reach forward and clasp the left wrist with the right hand around the left foot. Inhale, lift the head and chest. Exhale, place the chest on the left leg and the chin on the shin. Look toward the left foot—pada drishti. Remain here for five deep breaths.

Inhale, lift the head and chest, straightening the arms. Exhale, sit up. Place the palms of the hands on the floor on either side of the hips. Inhale, straighten the arms, lift the hips off of the floor, raise the left leg and touch the left shin to the chin. Exhale, swing back into Chaturanga Dandasana. Inhale, Urdhva Mukha Shvanasana. Exhale, Adho Mukha Shvanasana.

Jump forward with the right leg keeping it straight between the arms as you move the left leg to the left side of the left arm. Take hold of the left foot with the right hand and place the left lower leg behind the head. Straighten the right leg and flex the right foot. Place the palms of the hands together in front of the chest. Look toward the right foot—pada drishti. Remain here for five breaths.

Exhale, reach forward and clasp the right wrist with the left hand around the right foot. Inhale, lift the head and chest. Exhale, placing the chest on the right leg and the chin on the right shin. Look toward the right foot—pada drishti. Remain in this position for five breaths.

Inhale, lift the head and chest, straightening the arms. Exhale and sit up. Place the palms of the hands on the floor on either side of the hips. Inhale, straighten the arms, lift the hips up off of the floor, raise the right leg and touch the right shin to the chin. Exhale swing back into Chaturanga Dandasana. Inhale, Urdhva Mukha Shvanasana. Exhale, Adho Mukha Shvanasana.

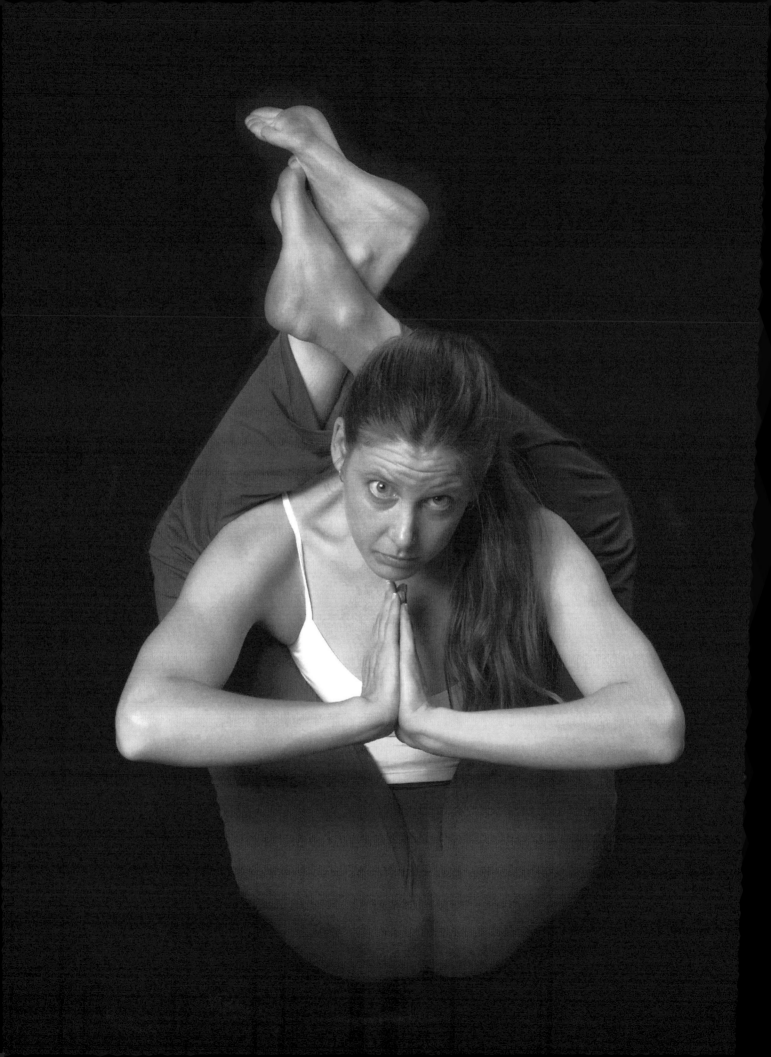

DWI PADA SHIRSHASANA

Jump forward around the arms. Sit down and place the left foot behind the head. Cross the right foot behind the left foot. Place the palms of the hands together and balance on the hips. While keeping the body steady, look towards the nose—nasa drishti—and take five deep breaths.

Then, place the palms of the hands on the floor next to the hips. While keeping the feet crossed, behind the head, straighten the arms in order to raise the hips up off of the floor. Inhale, straighten the legs into Tittibhasana. Exhale swing the feet back into Bakasana. Hop back into Chaturanga Dandasana. Inhale, Urdhva Mukha Shvanasana. Exhale, Adho Mukha Shvanasana.

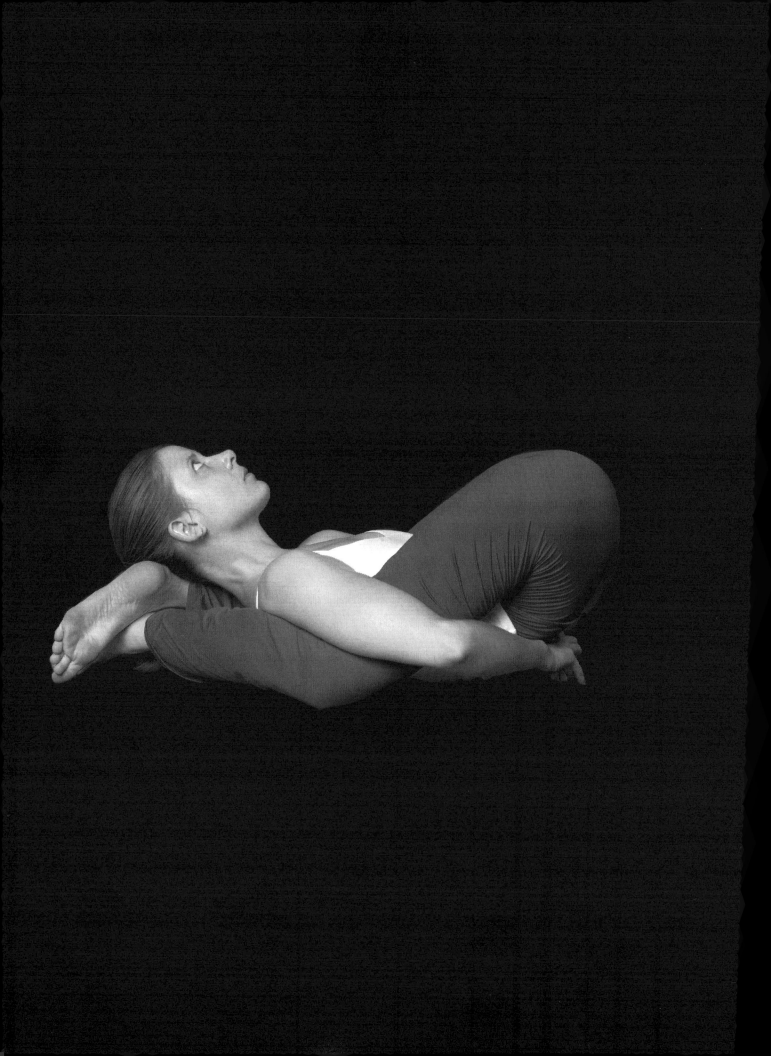

YOGANIDRASANA

Jump through the arms and exhale, lie down on the back.
Place the left foot behind the head. Then cross the right foot
behind the left foot. Tilt the head back and press the feet
into the floor with the head. Reach the arms back behind
the torso and grasp the left wrist with the right hand. Look
up into the forehead—ajna drishti—and breathe deeply for
five breaths.

Release the hands and uncross the feet. Swing the legs back
over the head, through Chakrasana into Chaturanga Dandasana. Inhale, Urdhva Mukha Shvanasana. Exhale, Adho
Mukha Shvanasana.

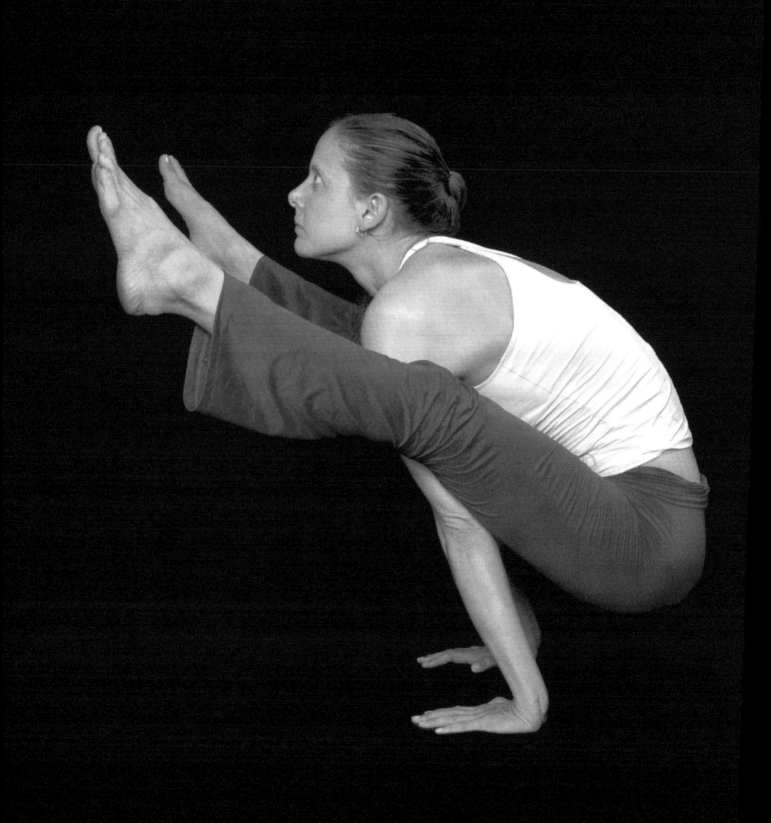

TITTIBHASANA A

A: Hop the legs forward onto the arms by engaging the abdominal muscles, arching the spine and raising the legs high. Land with the upper thighs high on the upper arms. Keep the arms straight throughout the movement. Drop the hips slightly, in order to straighten the legs at about a 30-degree angle to the floor. Point the toes, lift the head so that the chin is parallel to the floor, and look toward the nose—nasa drishti. Stay here for five deep breaths.

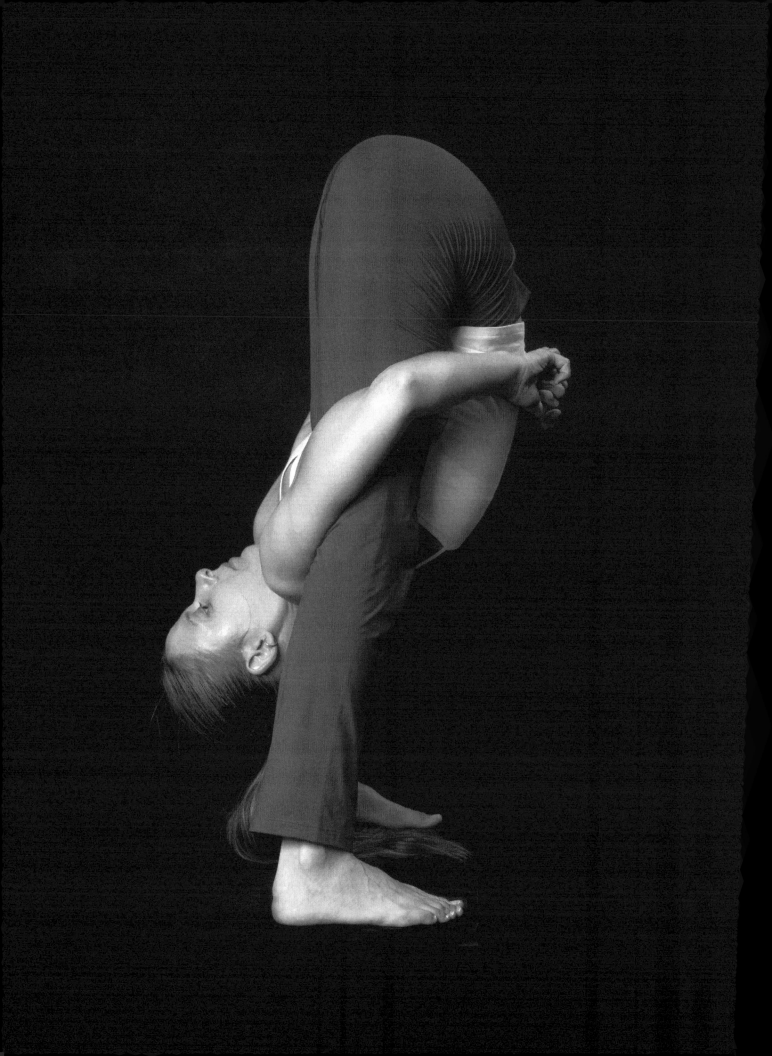

TITTIBHASANA B

B: Place feet on the floor, drop the torso and head down as you straighten the legs. Reach the arms through the legs and wrap them around the legs, grasping the left wrist with the right hand behind the back. Straighten the legs completely, lift the chin up to the chest and look towards the nose—nasa drishti. Remain here for five deep breaths.

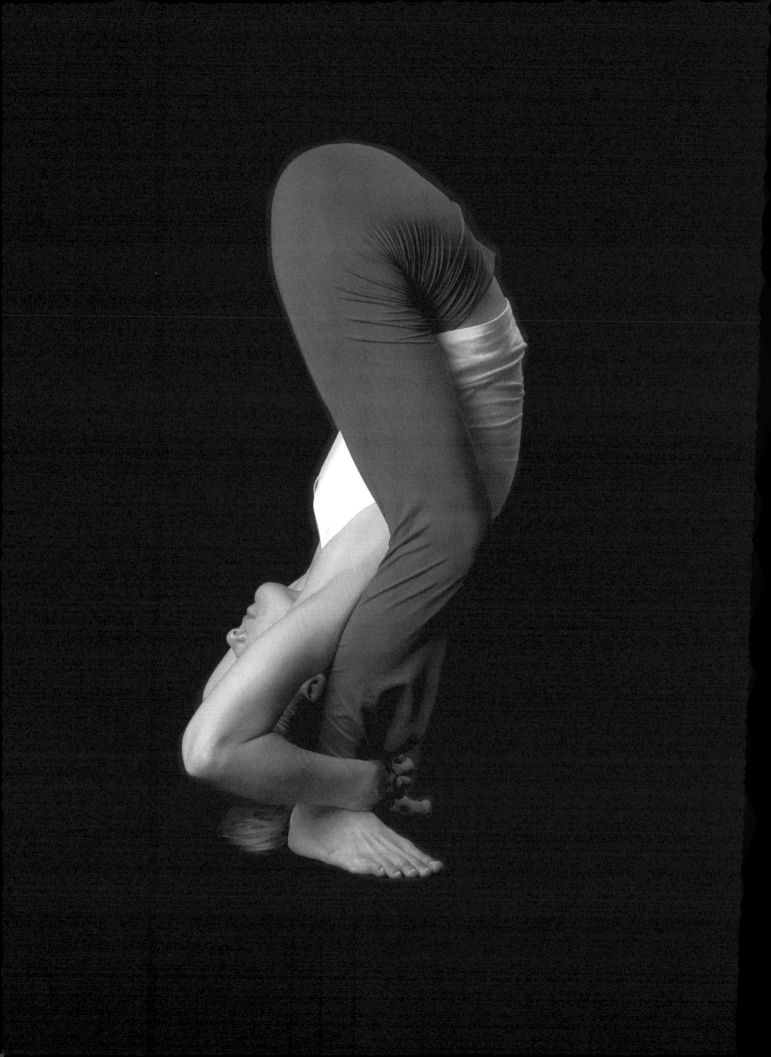

TITTIBHASANA C

C: Keeping the hands clasped behind the back, drop the head and look toward the floor. Take five steps forward and then five steps back, inhaling on one step and exhaling on the next.

Unclasp the hands and hold on to the ankles, dropping the torso down completely. Walk the legs toward each other behind the shoulders. Place the heels of the feet together allowing the toes to point slightly out to the sides. Clasp the hands around the ankles. Press into the feet and look towards the nose. Remain here for five deep breaths.

Place the palms of the hands on the floor, shoulder width apart on either side of the feet. Drop the hips and inhale, lift the legs back up into Tittibhasana A. Stay here in Tittibhasana A again for five deep breaths.

Exhale, swing the legs into Bakasana. Hop back into Chaturanga Dandasana. Inhale into Urdhva Mukha Shvanasana. Exhale into Adho Mukha Shvanasana.

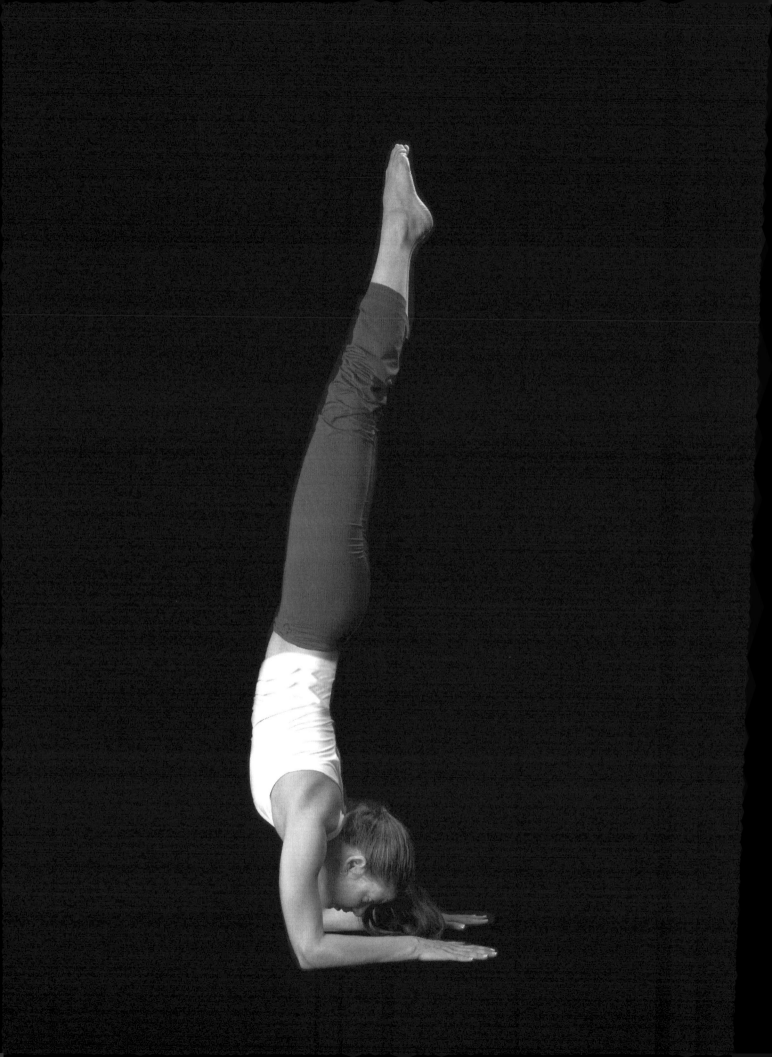

PINCHAMAYURASANA

Place the forearms on the floor, parallel to each other and shoulder width apart. Reach the chin forward. Hop the legs up above the head, keeping the legs straight. Balance on the forearms. Lift the ribcage above the elbows, by pressing the shoulders against the back. Position the body in a straight line, press the legs together gently and point the toes. Look towards the tip of the nose—nasa drishti—and breathe deeply for five breaths.

Press the forearms into the floor and quickly draw the ribcage down toward the elbows and hop onto the hands as you allow the body to lower down, moving it straight into Chaturanga Dandasana. Inhale, Urdhva Mukha Shvanasana. Exhale, Adho Mukha Shvanasana.

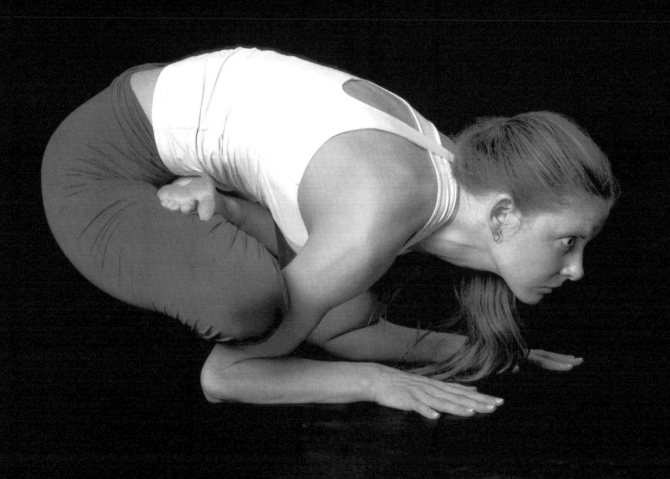

KARANDAVASANA

Lift back up into Pinchamayurasana. In Pinchamayurasana, cross the legs into Padmasana by placing the outside of the right foot against the front of the left hip, then reach the right knee up to the ceiling and place the outside of the left foot against the front of the right hip and reach the left knee up to the ceiling. Slowly lower the knees down and place them on the top of the upper arms, by folding at the hips and arching the spine tightly. Keep the hips raised, lift the head and look to the nose—nasa drishti.

Remain in Karandavasana for five deep breaths.

Slowly raise the hips up above the head. Extend the knees up to the ceiling. Press the shoulders against the back, to lift the ribcage above the elbows. Uncross and straighten the legs, extending them up to the ceiling into Pinchamayurasana. From here, hop into Chaturanga Dandasana. Inhale, Urdhva Mukha Shvanasana. Exhale, Adho Mukha Shvanasana.

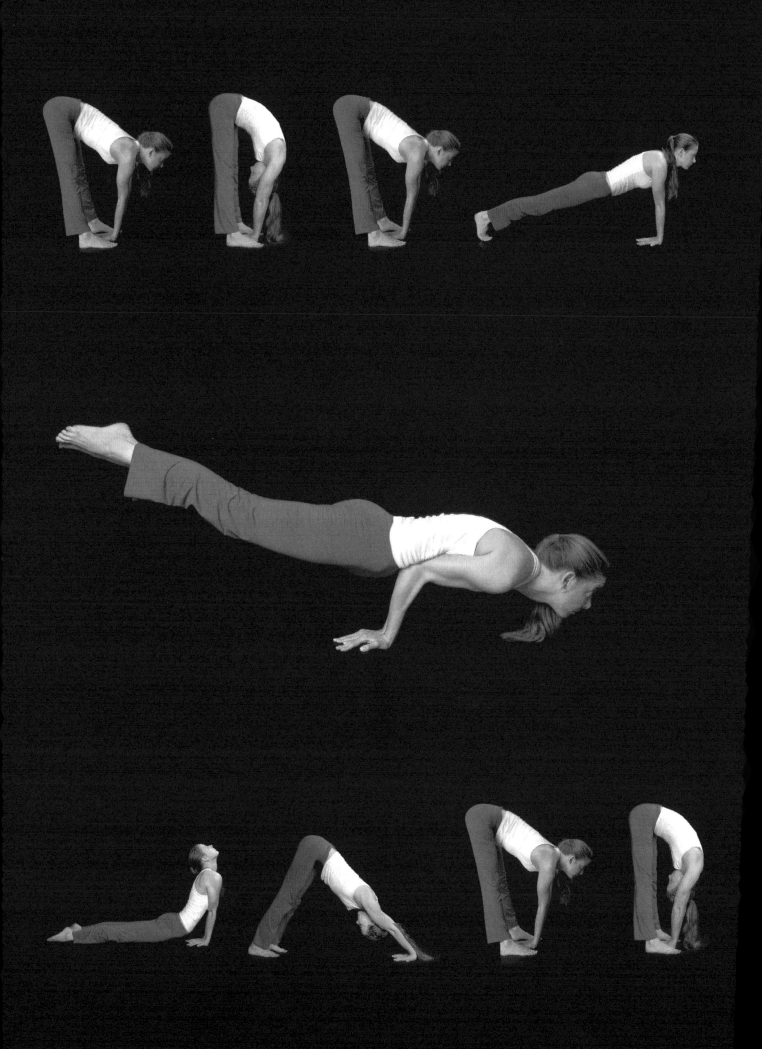

Hold the earth with both hands. Place the sides of the navel on the elbows. Rise high above the ground like a stick. This is Mayurasana.

Hatha Yoga Pradipika - Chapter 1, Verse 30

MAYURASANA

Inhale and hop forward between the hands and straighten the legs, spine and arms. Exhale, fold forward into Uttanasana. Inhale, raise the torso and reach the arms out the sides and up above the head until the palms of the hands touch. Tilt the head back and look towards the thumbs. Exhale, reach the arms out and down into Samastitihi. Hop the feet hip width apart. Exhale, bend forward and lower the arms, with the palms of the hands facing forward and upside down—the little finger sides of the hands touching. Place the palms of the hands on the floor next to each other with the fingers pointing back. Inhale, lift the head and straighten the arms. Exhale, hop the feet back and keep the arms straight, reaching a position in which the legs are straight and in line with the torso. Bend the elbows, push the body forward by rolling forward over the toes and place the navel onto the elbows. Lift the head, keep the legs straight, point the toes and raise the legs up away from the floor. Look to the nose—nasa drishti—and balance on the hands in Mayurasana for five deep breaths. Lower the toes to the floor, keeping the legs straight. Inhale, straighten the arms, lift the ribcage and arch the spine back. Exhale, lift the hips back and up. Drop the head between the arms and reach the heels down to the floor. Hop the feet forward around the hands. Inhale, lift the head until the arms straighten. Exhale, fold forward and pull the head back between the arms. Inhale, raise the torso, allowing the arms to drop down to the sides. Exhale hop the feet together into Samastitihi.

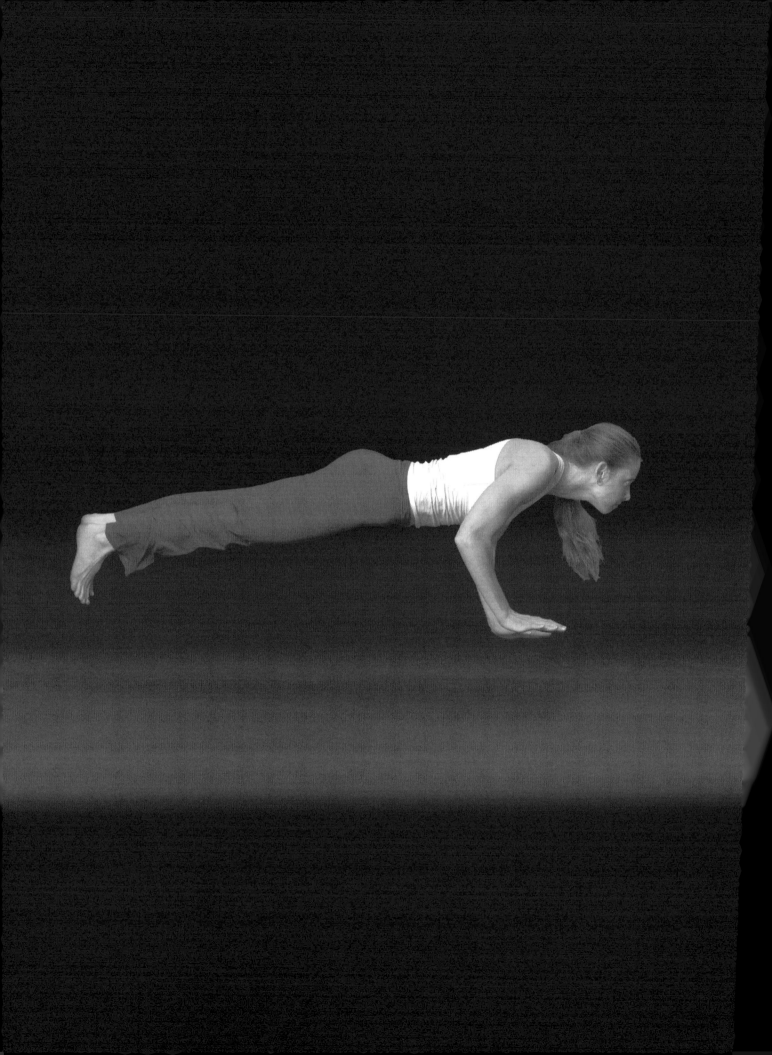

NAKRASANA

From Samastitihi, inhale, raise the arms above the head and tilt the head back. Exhale fold forward. Inhale raise the head, until the spine and arms straighten. Exhale hop back into Chaturanga Dandasana. Keep the body straight, extend the coccyx back and hop forward five times. Inhale as you lift the body and exhale as the body drops down. Then hop back five times.

Inhale, Urdhva Mukha Shvanasana. Exhale, Adho Mukha Shvanasana.

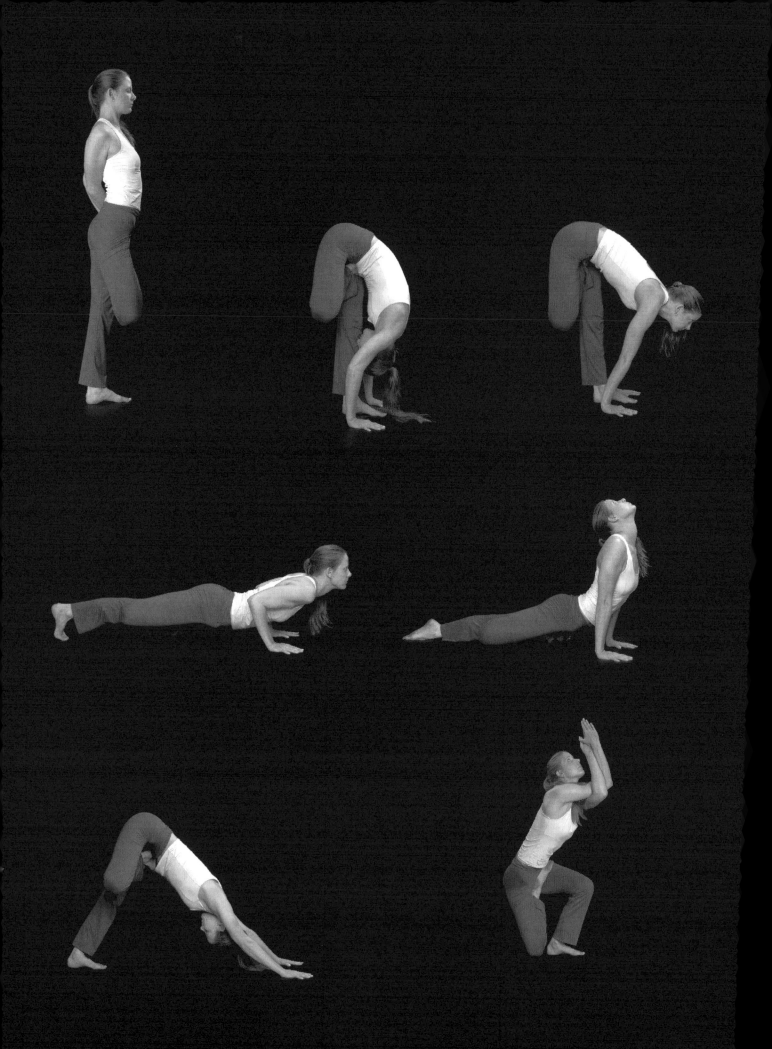

VATAYANASANA

Hop forward between the hands. Inhale and lift the head until the arms and spine straighten, keeping the finger tips in contact with the floor. Exhale, fold forward. Inhale, reach the arms out and up above the head. Tilt the head back and look to the thumbs. Exhale, reach the arms out and down and lower the chin into Samastitihi.

Stand on the left leg and raise the right foot into Ardha Padmasana, by placing the outside of the right foot against the front of the left hip. Reach the right arm behind the back and take hold of the right big toe, with the first two fingers and thumb of the right hand. Exhale fold forward and place the palm of the left hand on the floor to the left of the left foot and then release the right arm and place the palm of the right hand on the floor to the right of the left foot. Inhale raise the head, until the arms and spine straighten while keeping the fingertips in contact with the floor. Exhale, hop the left foot back into Chaturanga Dandasana and extend the right knee back, keeping it in Ardha Padmasana. Inhale, reach the rib cage forward into

Urdhva Mukha Shvanasana and exhale, lift the hips back and up into Adho Mukha Shvanasana with the right leg in Ardha Padmasana. Hop the left foot forward between the hands. Rotate the left foot to the left and place the right knee on the floor to the right of the left heel. Raise the torso and balance on the left foot and right knee. With bent elbows, cross the right elbow over the left upper arm, wrap the right forearm out and around the left forearm and place the palms of the hands together, so that the fingers point up to the ceiling. Then raise the arms, tilt the head back and look up to the thumbs. Balance in Vatayanasana on the left side for five deep breaths.

Release the arms and place the palms of the hands on the floor, shoulder width apart in front of the left foot and right knee. Exhale, hop the left foot back into Chaturanga Dandasana and extend the left knee back, keeping the right foot in Ardha Padmasana. Inhale, Urdhva Mukha Shvanasana and exhale Adho Mukha Shvanasana, with the right leg in Ardha Padmasana. Then step the right foot down

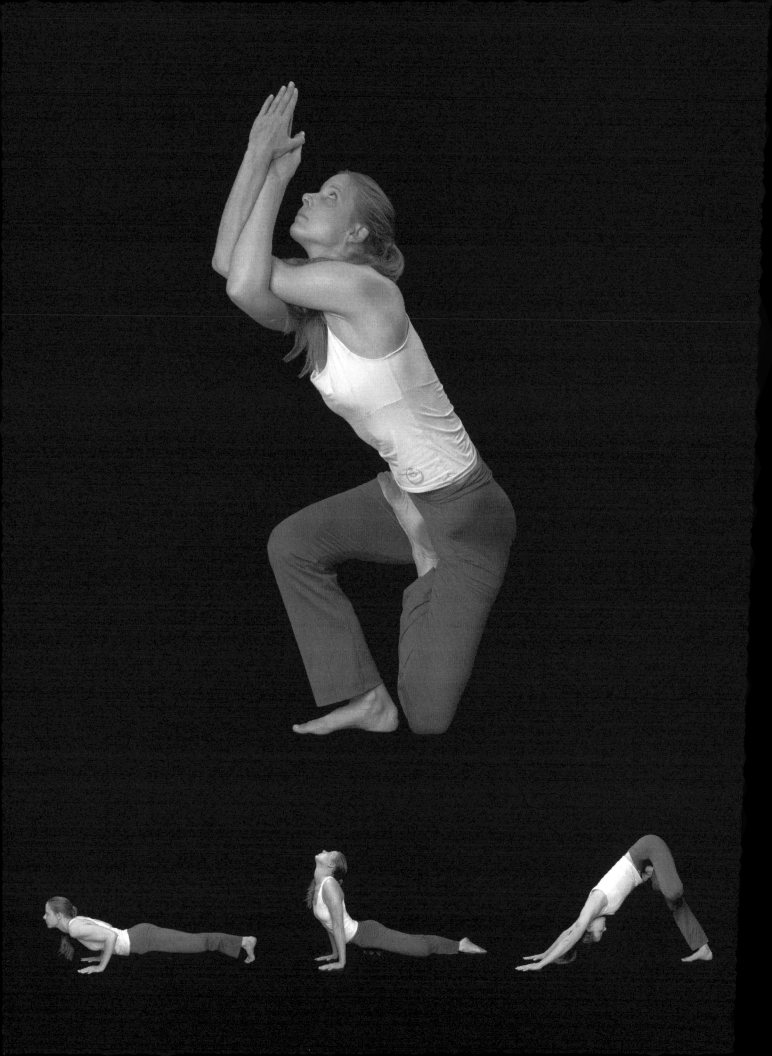

VATAYANASANA ...continued

into Adho Mukha Shvanasana and place the outside of the left foot into Ardha Padmasana, in the crease of the right hip. Then hop the right foot forward between the hands. Rotate the right foot to the right and place the left knee on the floor to the left of the right heel. Raise the torso and balance on the right foot and left knee. With bent elbows, cross the left elbow over the right upper arm, wrap the left forearm out and around the right forearm, and place the palms of the hands together so that the fingers point up to the ceiling. Then raise the arms and tilt the head, looking up to the thumbs. Balance in Vatayanasana on the right side for five deep breaths.

Release the arms and place the palms of the hands on the floor, shoulder width apart in front of the right foot and left

knee. Exhale hop the right foot back into Chaturanga Dandasana and extend the right knee back, keeping the left foot in Ardha Padmasana. Inhale, Urdhva Mukha Shvanasana and exhale Adho Mukha Shvansana, with the left leg in Ardha Padmasana. Hop the right foot forward between the hands. Inhale raise the head, until the arms and spine straighten, keeping the fingertips in contact with the floor. Exhale fold forward, press the palm of the right hand into the floor and reach the left arm behind the back, taking hold of the left big toe with first two fingers and the thumb of the left hand. Inhale, raise the torso, back up to standing and place the right hand on the right hip. Exhale, release the grip of the left hand on the left big toe and place the left foot on the floor next to the right foot into Samastitihi.

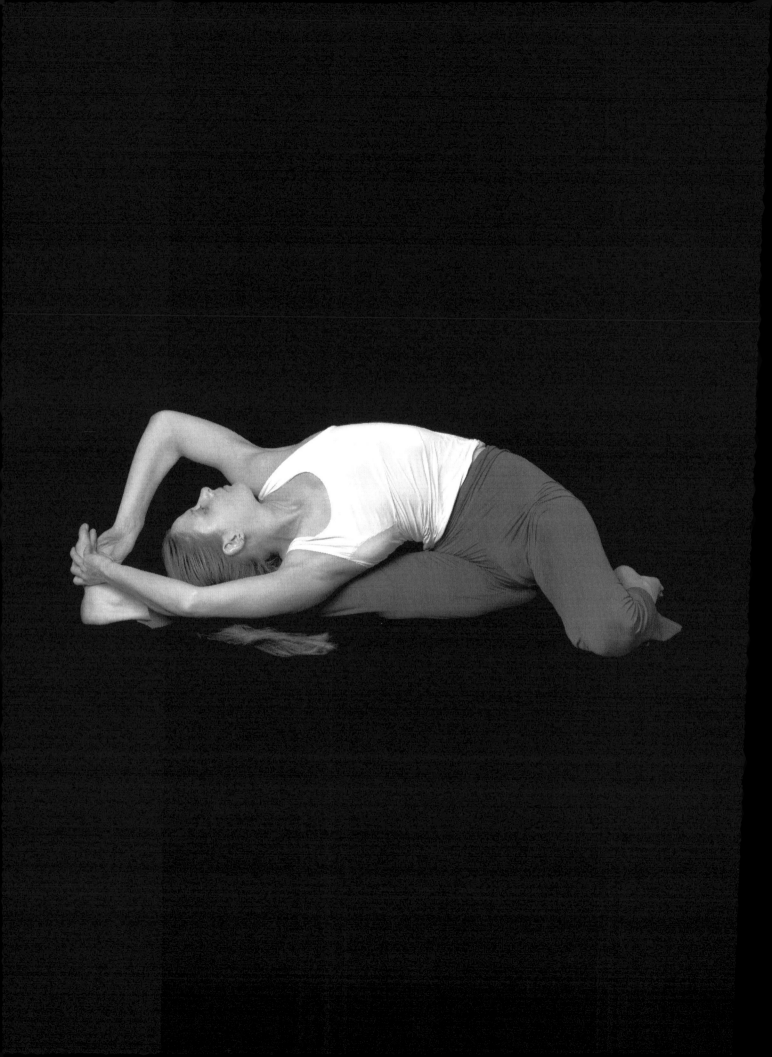

PARIGHASANA

Inhale and reach the arms out and up above the head. Tilt the head back and look up to the thumbs. Exhale, fold forward into Uttanasana and place the palms of the hands on the floor on either side of the feet. Inhale, raise the head until the spine and arms straighten while keeping the finger tips in contact with the floor. Exhale, Chaturanga Dandasana. Inhale, Urdhva Mukha Shvanasana. Exhale Adho Mukha Shvanasana. Hop through the arms, with the left leg bent so that the left knee extends forward and the left toes point back. The right leg remains straight as it reaches through the arms and extends 90 degrees to the right. The hips land on the floor between the hands. Inhale, place the palms of the hands on the hips and lift the rib cage. Then exhale, tilt the torso to the right, reach the right arm forward with the palm of the right hand facing up, twist the torso to the left, so that the rib cage faces up to the ceiling. Reach the right hand up and take hold of the inside of the right foot with the little finger side of the hand facing up. Reach the left hand to the left and up over the head to take hold of the outside of the right foot; keep the little finger side of the hand facing up. Then draw the left elbow down to the left and rotate the head to the left, until the back of the head rests on the lower leg and look to the nose—nasa drishti. Remain in Parighasana on the right side for five deep breaths.

Release the hands and inhale, raise the torso back up to a seated position. Press the palms of the hands into the floor on either side of the left thigh, shoulder width apart, and hop back into Chaturanga Dandasana. Inhale, Urdhva Mukha Shvanasana. Exhale, Adho Mukha Shvanasana.

Hop through the arms for Parighasana on the left side, by extending the right knee forward with the right toes pointing back and extending the left leg, keeping it straight, through the arms and reaching it 90 degrees to the left. Inhale, place the palms of the hands on the hips and lift the rib cage. Exhale, tilt the torso to the left and rotate it to the right. Reach the left hand up over the head and take hold of the inside of the left foot with the left hand and reach the right arm to the right and up over the head and take hold of the outside of the left foot with the right hand. Draw the right elbow down to the right, rotate the head to the right and look to the nose—nasa drishti. Stay in Parighasana on the left side for five deep breaths.

Inhale, release the hands and sit up. Exhale, press the palms of the hands into the floor on either side of the right thigh and hop back into Chaturanga Dandasana. Inhale, Urdhva Mukha Shvanasana. Exhale, Adho Mukha Shvanasana.

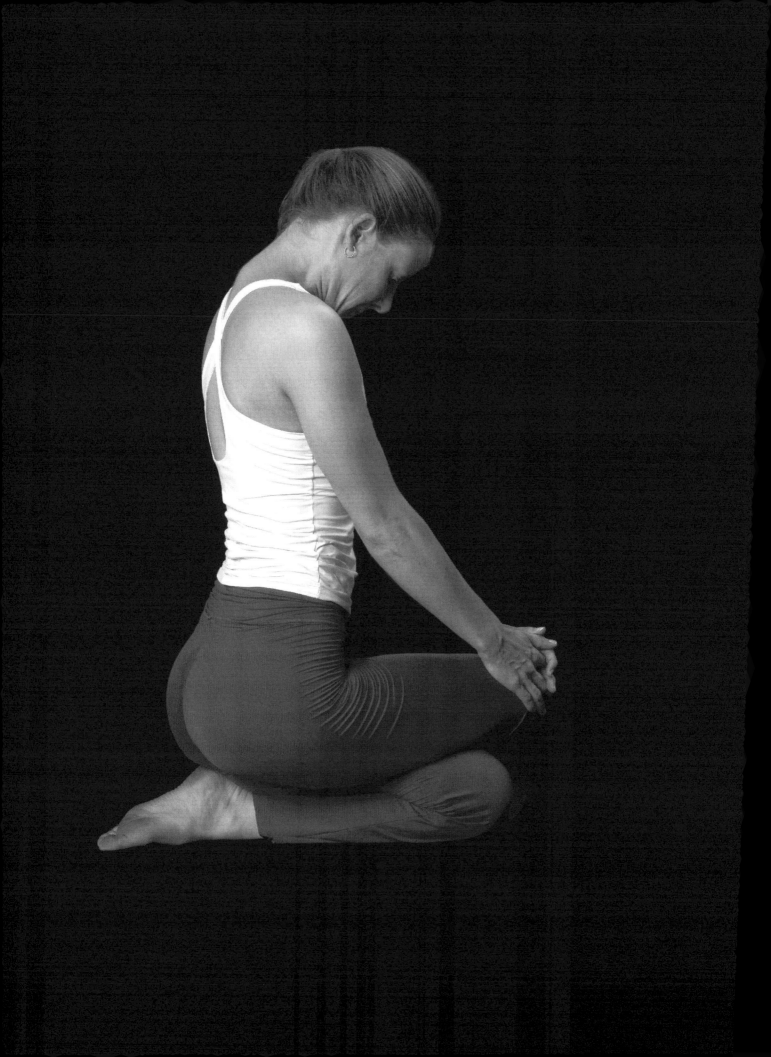

GOMUKHASANA A

Hop forward with the knees bent, the right leg crossed over the left leg and the toes pointing back. Sit down on the heels. Reach the arms forward, keeping them straight, and hold onto the right knee with both hands, by placing one hand on top of the other hand. Lift the ribcage, press the chin against the sternum and look toward the nose. Take five deep breaths in Gomukhasana A on the right side.

Raise the right arm above the head, bend the right elbow and lower the right hand down the back between the shoulder blades. Reach the left arm behind the back, bend the left elbow. Reach the left hand up to the right hand and take hold of the fingers of the right hand with the fingers of the left hand. Then, tilt the head back and look up to the ceiling—urdhva drishti. Stay in Gomukhasana B on the right side for five deep breaths.

Release the arms, press the palms of the hands into the floor on either side of the knees and hop back into Chaturanga Dandasana. Inhale, Urdhva Mukha Shvanasana. Exhale, Adho Mukha Shvanasana. Then hop forward with the knees bent, the left leg crossed over the right leg, the lower legs together and the toes pointing back. Sit down on the heels. Reach the arms forward, keeping them straight, and hold onto the left knee with both hands, by placing one hand on top of the other hand. Lift the ribcage, press the chin against the sternum and look towards the nose. Take five deep breaths in Gomukhasana A on the left side.

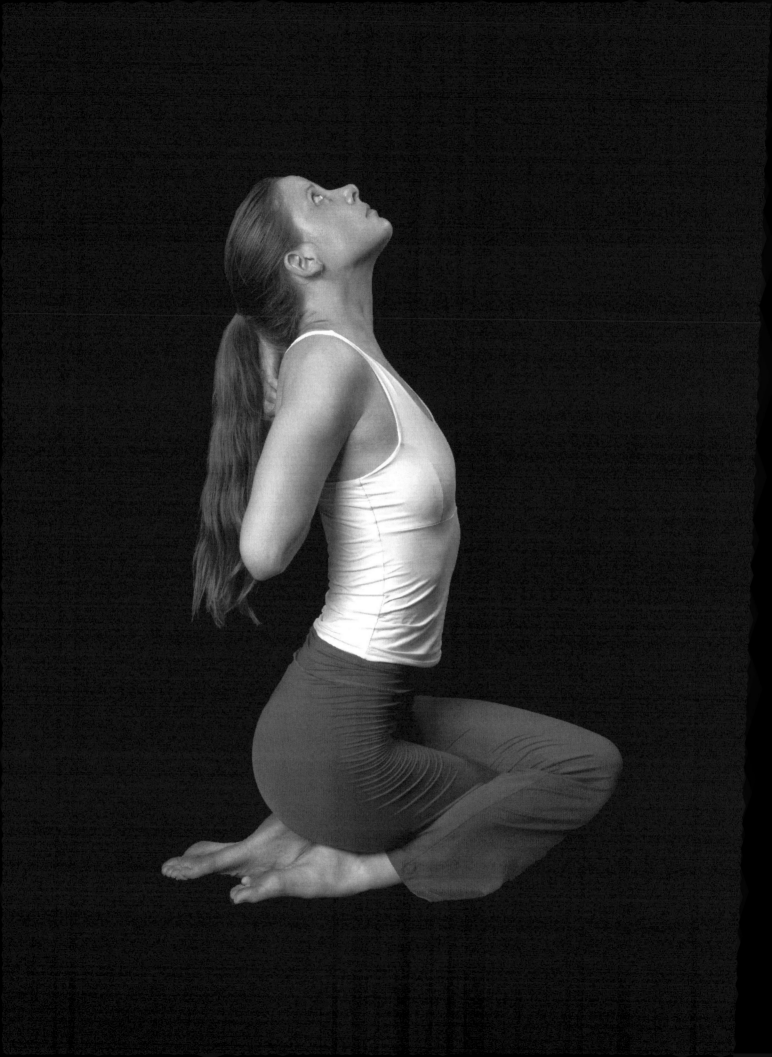

GOMUKHASANA B

Then raise the left arm above the head, bend the left elbow and lower the left hand down the back between the shoulder blades. Reach the right arm behind the back, bend the right elbow, reach the right hand up to the left hand and take hold of the fingers of the left hand with the fingers of the right hand. Tilt the head back and look up to the ceiling (Urdhva Drishti). Remain in Gomukhasana B on the left side for five deep breaths.

Release the arms, press the palms of the hands into the floor on either side of the knees and hop back into Chaturanga Dandasana. Inhale into Urdhva Mukha Shvanasana. Exhale into Adho Mukha Shvanasana.

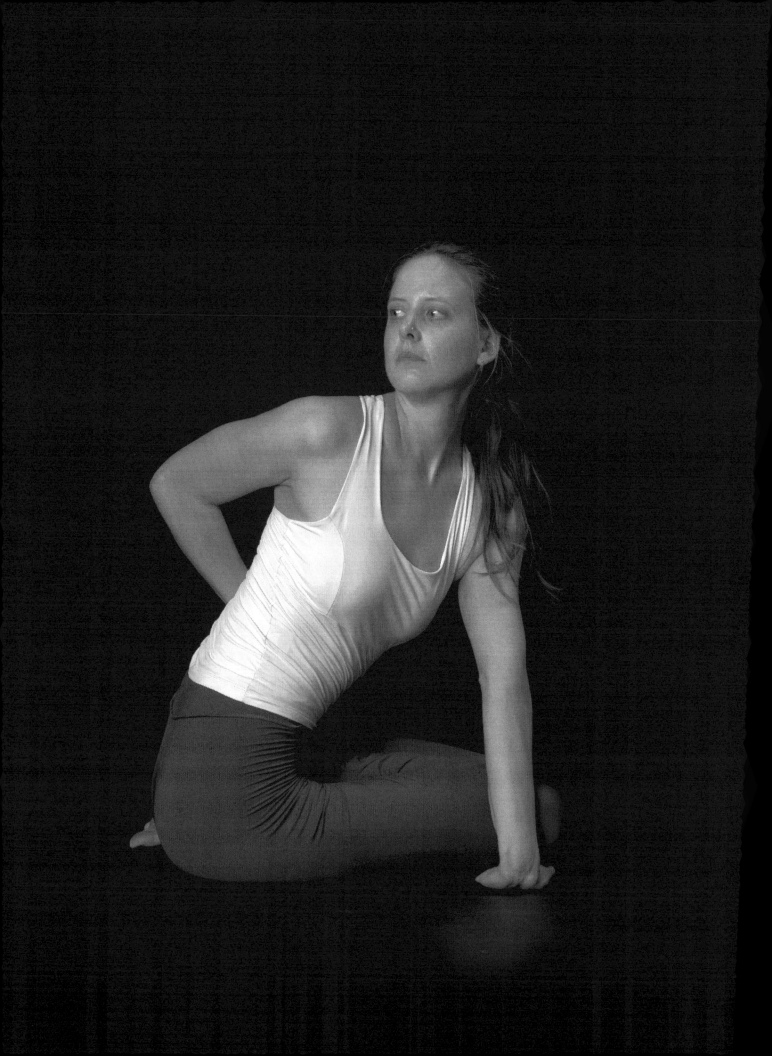

SUPTA URDHVA VAJRASANA

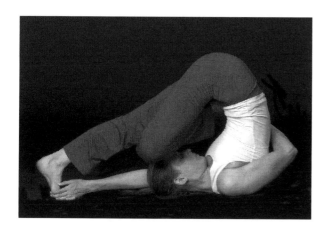

Jump through the arms and lie down on the back. Raise the legs, keeping them straight, and reach them over the head, by raising the hips and shifting the weight of the body into the shoulders and back of the head. Then bend the right leg and place the right foot into the crease of the left hip to achieve Ardha Padmasana. Reach the right arm behind the back and take hold of the right big toe with the first two fingers and thumb of the right hand. Then, reach the left arm over the head to the inside of the left foot, with the palm of the left hand facing up. Take hold of the inside of the left foot by raising the

thumb of the left hand. Exhale, rock up to sitting and keep hold of right big toe with the right hand. Bend the left leg by pulling the left toes back with the left hand and extend the left knee forward, next to the right knee.

Pull the knees together by flexing the right foot and place the palm of the left hand underneath the right knee with the fingers of the left hand pointing to the left - do this by rotating the left arm externally and keeping it straight. Keeping hold of the right big toe with the right hand, rotate the torso and head to the right. Look to the right—parshva drishti—and remain in Supta Urdhva Vajrasana to the right for five deep breaths.

Release the arms and torso and untwist the torso back to center. Press the palms of the hands into the floor on either side of the thighs and hop back into Chaturanga

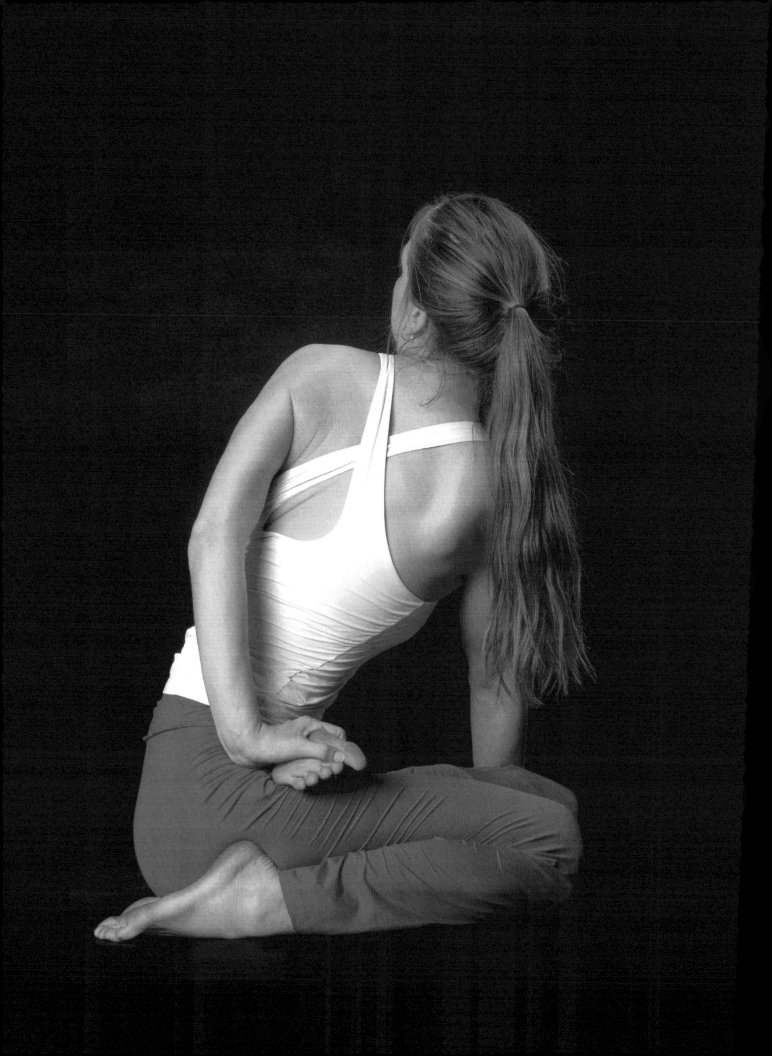

SUPTA URDHVA VAJRASANA ... continued

Dandasana. Inhale, Urdhva Mukha Shvanasana. Exhale, Adho Mukha Shvanasana. Jump through and lie down on the back. Reach the legs over the head, keeping them straight until the toes touch the floor. Place the left foot into the crease of the right hip. Reach the left arm behind the back and take hold of the left big toe with the first two fingers and the thumb of the left hand. Then, reach the right arm over the head to the inside of the right foot, with the palm of the right hand facing up. Take hold of the inside of the right foot by raising the right thumb. Exhale, rock up to sitting, keep hold of the left big toe with the left hand and bend the right leg by pulling the right toes back with the right hand. Extend the right knee forward next to the left knee.

Pull the knees together by flexing the left foot, and place the palm of the right hand underneath the left knee. The fingers of the right hand are pointing to the right through a rotation of the right arm externally while keeping it straight.

Keeping hold of the left big toe with the left hand, rotate the torso and head to the left. Look to the left—parshva drishti—and remain in Supta Urdhva Vajrasana to the left for five deep breaths.

Release the arms and torso and untwist back to center. Press the palms of the hands into the floor on either side of the thighs and hop back into Chaturanga Dandasana. Inhale, Urdhva Mukha Shvanasana. Exhale, Adho Mukha Shvanasana.

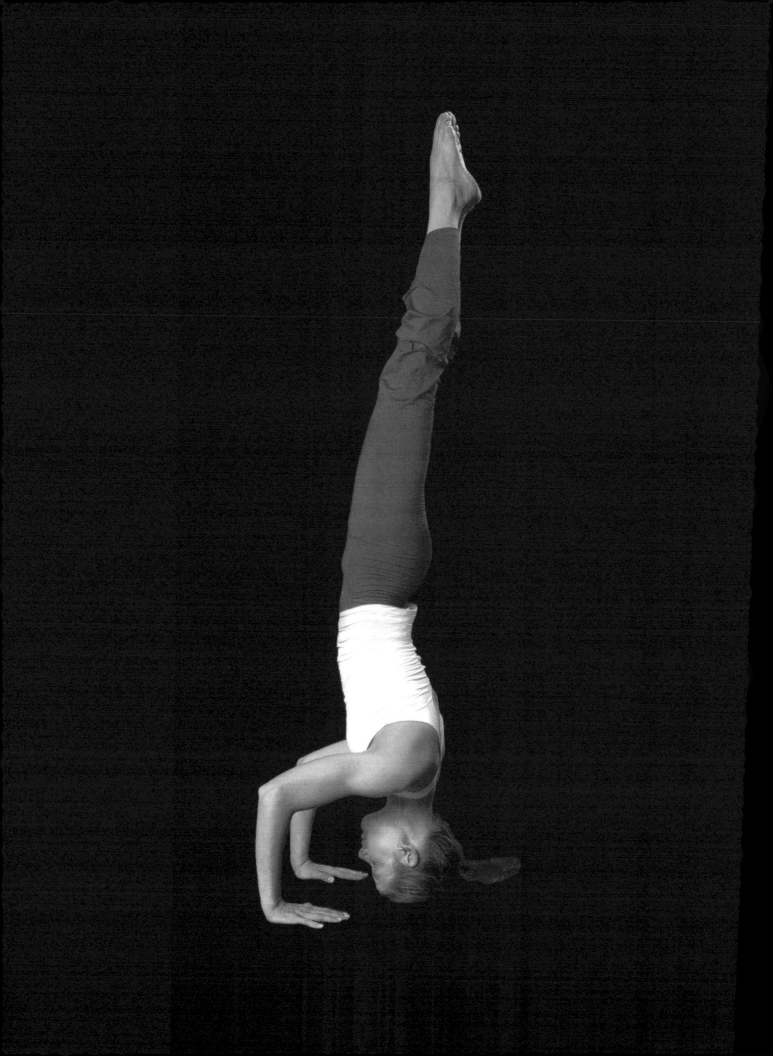

MUKHTA HASTA SHIRSHASANA A

Come down onto the knees. Place the top of the head on the floor in front of the hands, creating an equilateral triangle with the hands, forearms and head. Raise the hips above the head, by pressing the toes and elbows into the floor and bringing the legs together and straight. Then, inhale and raise the legs, keeping them straight above the head and in line with the torso. Point the toes, look towards the nose— nasa drishti—and stay in Mukhta Hasta Shirshasana A for five deep breaths.

Keeping the body straight, drop down, lift the head and pull the rib cage forward into Chaturanga Dandasana on the exhale. Inhale, Urdhva Mukha Shvanansana. Exhale, Adho Mukha Shvanasana.

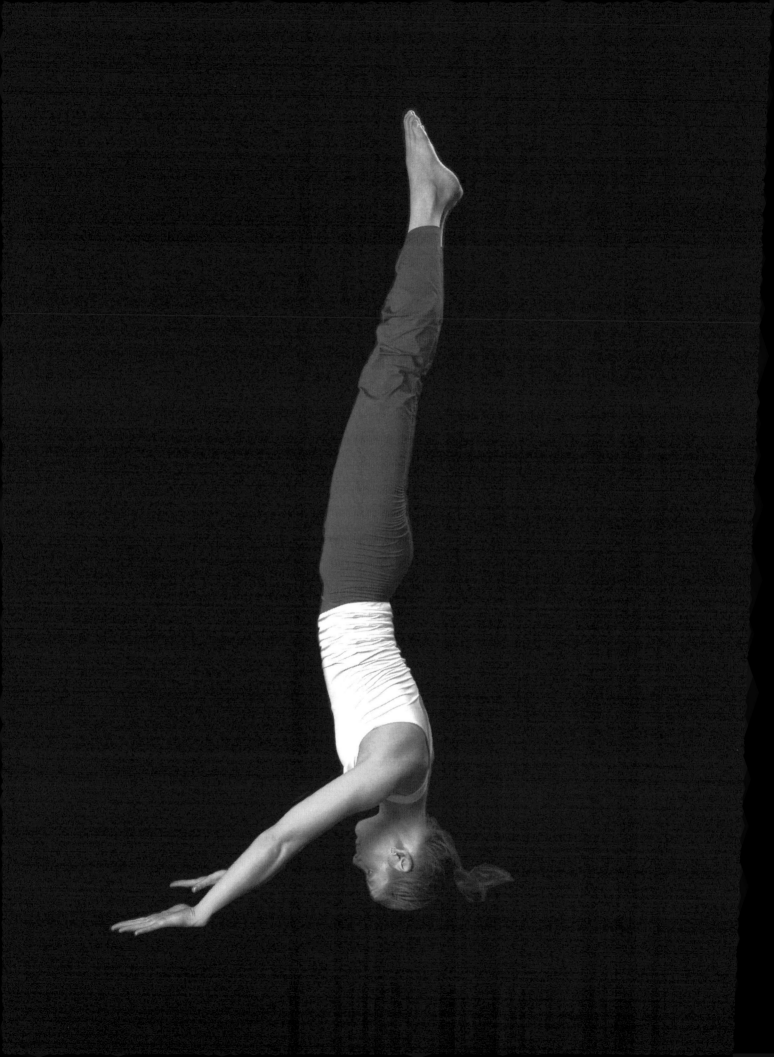

MUKHTA HASTA SHIRSHASANA B

Drop down onto the knees. Place the top of the head on
the floor in front of the hands and forearms. Raise the hips
above the head by pressing the toes and elbows into the
floor and bringing the legs together and straightening them.
Reach the arms toward the feet and press the backs of the
hands into the floor with straight arms shoulder width apart.
Then, inhale and raise the legs keeping them straight above
the head in line with the torso. Point the toes, look towards
the tip of the nose—nasa drishti—and stay in Mukhta Hasta
Shirshasana B for five deep breaths.

Keeping the body straight, drop down, lift the head and
pull the rib cage forward into Chaturanga Dandasana on the
exhale. Inhale, Urdhva Mukha Shvanasana. Exhale, Adho
Mukha Shvanasana.

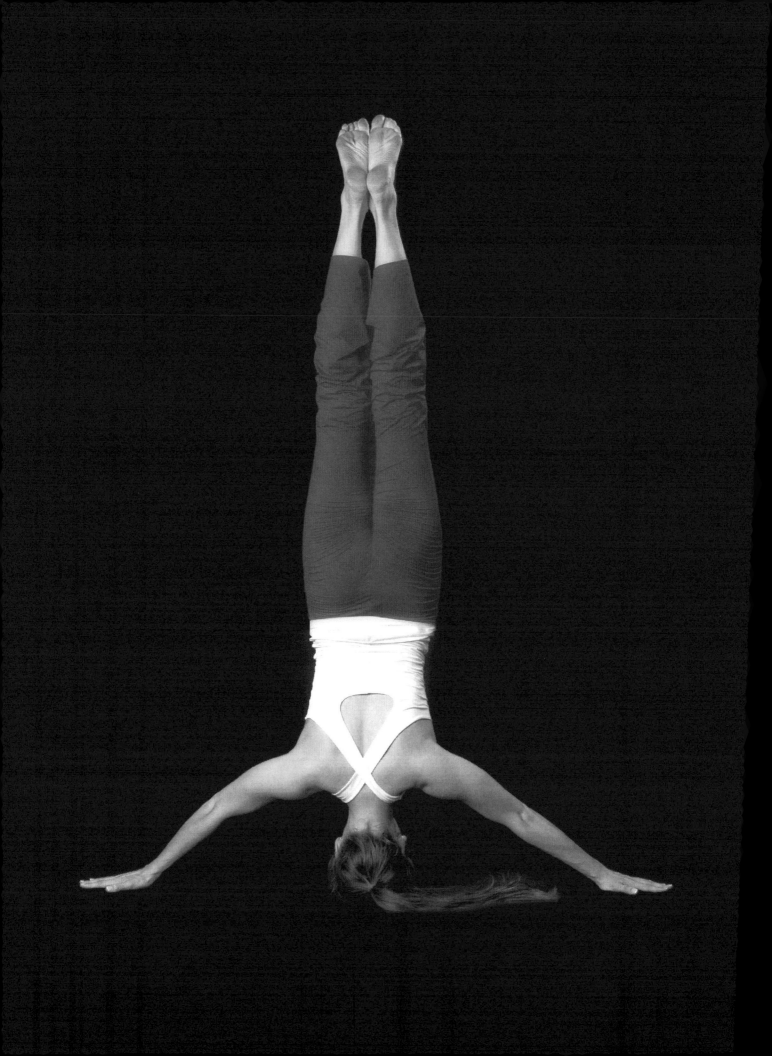

MUKHTA HASTA SHIRSHASANA C

Drop down onto the knees. Place the top of the head on the floor in front of the hands. Raise the hips above the head by pressing the toes and elbows into the floor and bringing the legs together and straight. Reach the arms out to the sides and place the palms of the hands on the floor on either side of the head. On the inhaling breath, raise the legs and keep them straight above the head in line with the torso. Point the toes, look at the nose——nasa drishti–and balance in Mukhta Hasta Shirshasana C for five deep breaths. Keeping the body straight, drop down, lift the head and pull the rib cage forward into Chaturanga Dandasana on the exhale. Inhale, into Urdhva Mukha Shvanasana. Exhale, Adho Mukha Shvanasana.

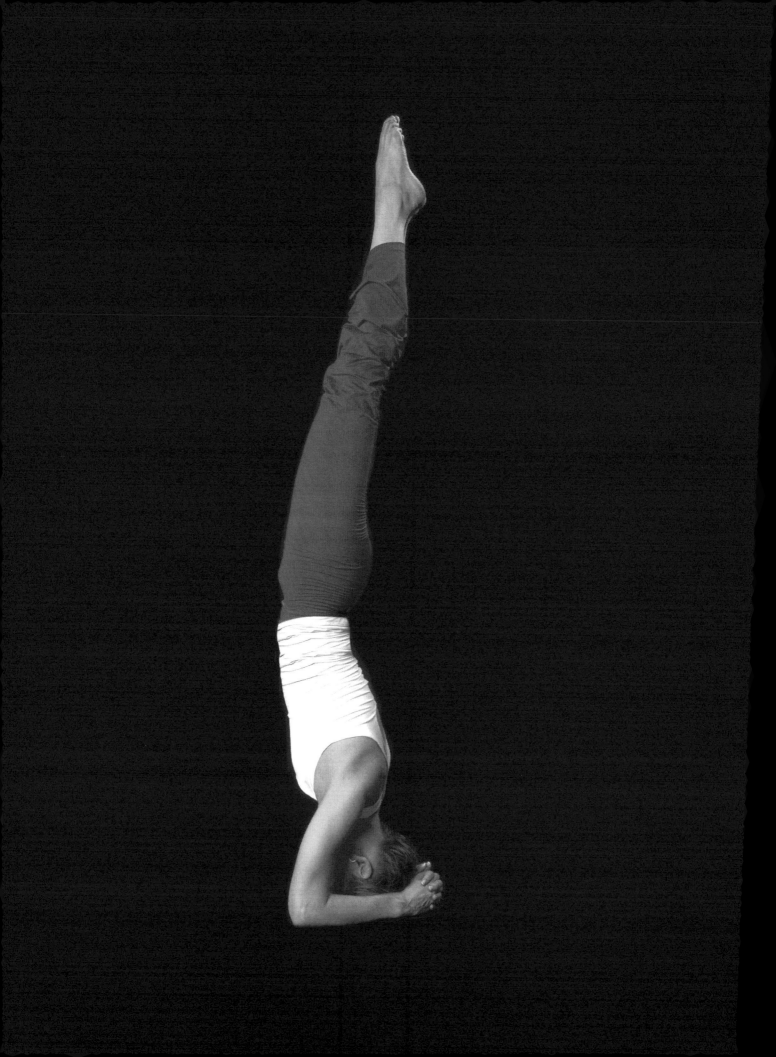

BADDHA HASTA SHIRSHASANA A

Drop down onto the knees. Interlace the fingers, and place the forearms on the floor with the elbows shoulder width apart. Place the top of the head on the floor, with the back of the head resting against the palms of the hands. Raise the hips above the head by pressing the toes and elbows into the floor and bringing the legs together as you straighten them. On the inhale, raise the legs keeping them straight above the head in line with the torso. Point the toes, look at the nose—nasa drishti—and balance in Baddha Hasta Shirshasana A for five deep breaths. Keeping the body straight, drop down and lift the head, pulling the rib cage forward into Chaturanga Dandasana on the exhale. Inhale into Urdhva Mukha Shvanasana. Exhale Adho Mukha Shvanasana.

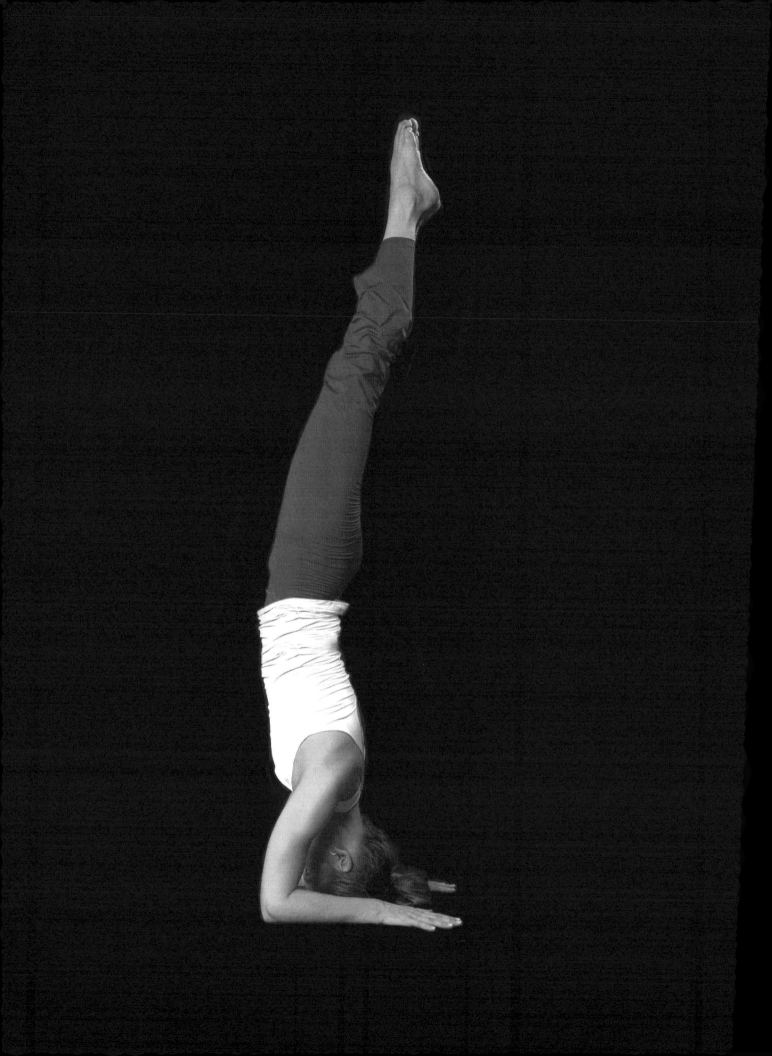

BADDHA HASTA SHIRSHASANA B

Drop down onto the knees. Place the forearms on the floor with the palms of the hands facing down, shoulder width apart, parallel to each other. Place the top of the head on the floor between the forearms. Raise the hips above the head, by pressing the toes and elbows into the floor and bringing the legs together as you straighten them. On the inhaling breath, raise the legs, keeping them straight above the head in line with the torso. Point the toes, look at the nose—nasa drishti—and balance in Baddha Hasta Shirshasana B for five deep breaths. Keeping the body straight, drop down and lift the head, pulling the rib cage forward into Chaturanga Dandasana on the exhale. Inhale, Urdhva Mukha Shvanasana. Exhale, Adho Mukha Shvanasana.

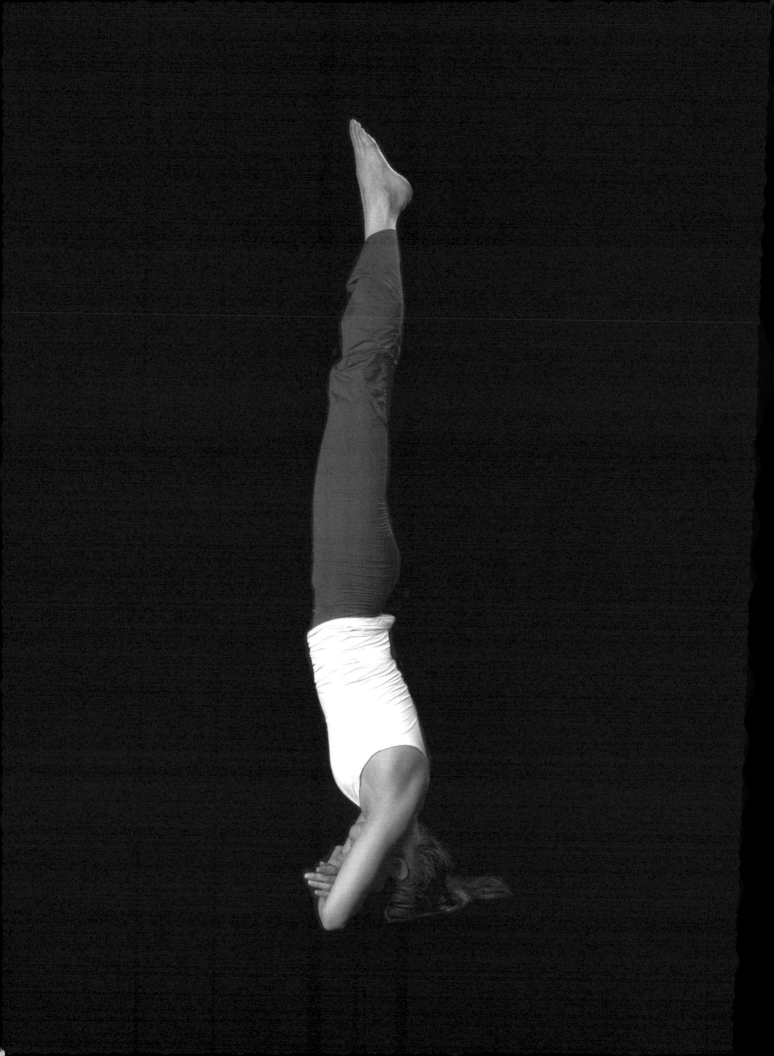

BADDHA HASTA SHIRSHASANA C

Drop down onto the knees. Cross the forearms, placing the hands in the crease of the elbows. Place the forearms on the floor and the top of the head on the floor in front of the forearms. Raise the hips above the head by pressing the toes and elbows into the floor and bringing the legs together as you straighten them. On the inhaling breath, raise the legs straight above the head in line with the torso. Point the toes and look at the nose—nasa drishti. Balance in Baddha Hasta Shirshasana C for five deep breaths. Keeping the body straight, drop down and lift the head while pulling the rib cage forward into Chaturanga Dandasana on the exhale. Inhale, Urdhva Mukha Shvanasana. Exhale, Adho Mukha Shvanasana.

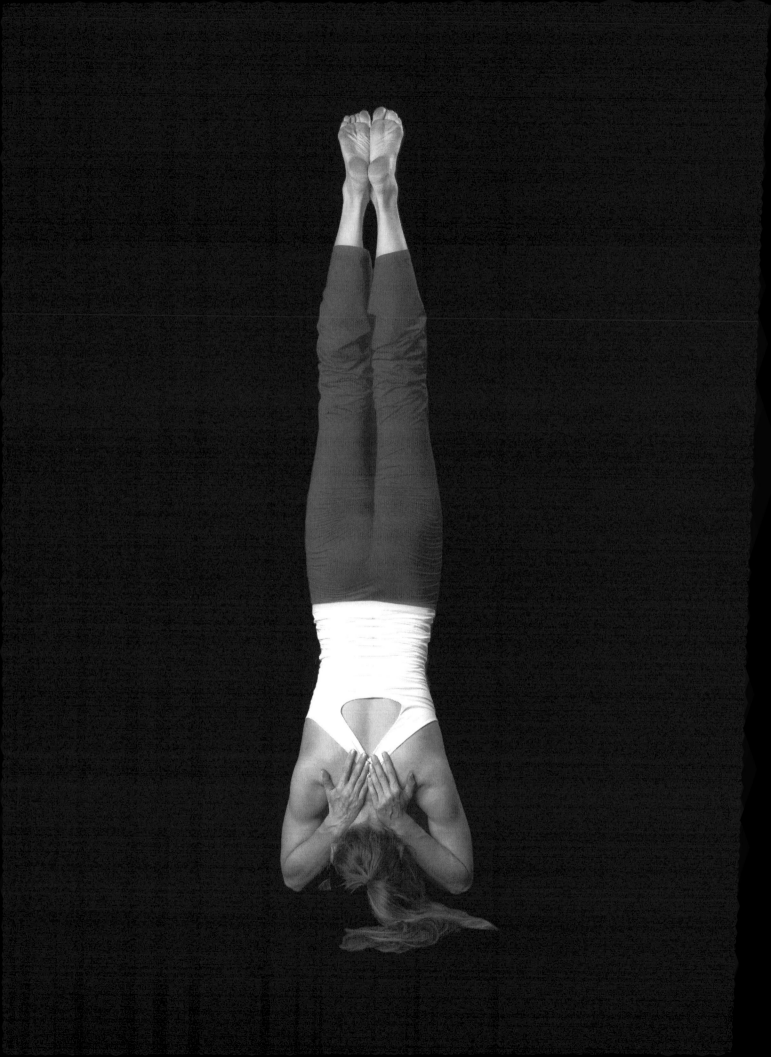

BADDHA HASTA SHIRSHASANA D

Drop down onto the knees. Place the top of the head onto the floor. Bend the elbows and press them into the floor, shoulder width apart and a few inches in front of the face. Place the palms of the hands on the shoulders. On the inhaling breath, raise the legs keeping them straight above the head in line with the torso. Point the toes and look at the nose—nasa drishti. Balance in Baddha Hasta Shirshasana D for five deep breaths. Keeping the body straight, drop down and lift the head, pulling the rib cage forward into Chaturanga Dandasana on the exhale. Inhale into Urdhva Mukha Shvanasana. Exhale Adho Mukha Shvanasana.

The Finishing Sequence of asanas are practiced after completing the asanas of either the primary or intermediate series. When starting the practice with the primary series, the finishing asanas are added after the practitioner has completed the asanas up to Navasana. When the practitioner has completed the asanas of the primary series, the finishing asanas are practiced after Setu Bandhasana. When practicing the intermediate series, the finishing asanas are practiced after Baddha Hasta Shirshasana.

FINISHING ASANAS

The finishing asanas begin with Urdhva Dhanurasana, the upward facing bow posture. After practicing Urdhva Dhanurasana, Paschimottanasana is practiced for ten breaths. At this stage the breath is slowed down and the nervous system is calmed down in preparation for the fundamental asanas of the finishing sequence, which include sarvangasana (shoulderstand), Matsyasana (fish posture), Shirshasana (head stand), Padmasana (lotus posture) and Shavasana(corpse posture), the final relaxation at the end of the practice.

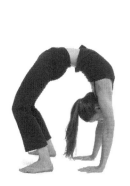

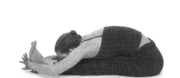

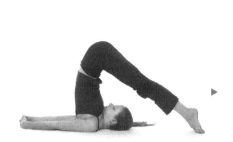

URDHVA
DHANURASANA   PASCHIMOTTANASANA   SARVANGASANA   HALASANA

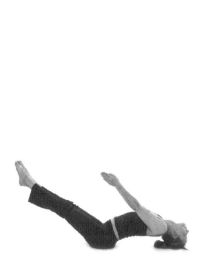

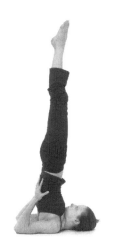

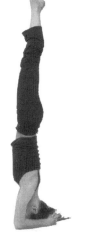

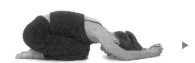

UTTANAPADASANA   A   B   BALASANA

SHIRSHASANA

ASHTANGA YOGA

FINISHING ASANAS

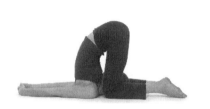

KARNAPIDASANA

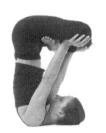

URDHVAPADMASANA

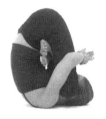

PINDASANA

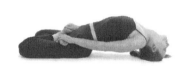

MATSYASANA

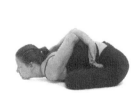

YOGAMUDRA

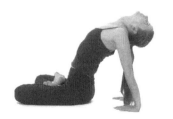

YOGAMUDRA2

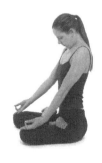

PADMASANA

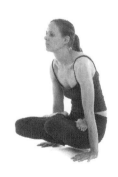

UTHPLUTIHI

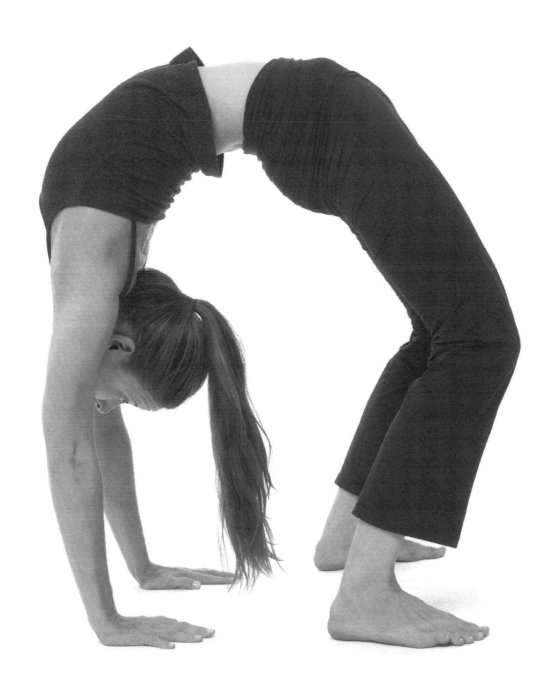

URDHVA DHANURASANA

From Adho Mukha Shvanasana, hop through the arms and lie down on the back. Bend the knees completely and place the soles of the feet on the floor, slightly wider than hip width apart, with the toes pointing forward. Then, place the palms of the hands on the floor on either side of the head, shoulder width apart, with the elbows pointing up and the fingers pointing in the direction of the feet.

Inhale, press into the hands and feet, raise the hips and spine up to the ceiling and allow the head to drop down between the arms. Look toward the nose—nasa drishti—and stay in Urdhva Dhanurasana for five breaths.

Exhale, lower the torso back down to the floor, lift the head and place the back of the head on the floor. Inhale, press back up into Urdhva Dhanurasana. Walk the hands closer to the feet to deepen the arch and remain here for another five deep breaths.

Exhale and lower the torso down to the floor, lift the head and place the back of the head on the floor. Inhale, lift up into Urdhva Dhanurasana a third time and breathe deeply for five breaths.

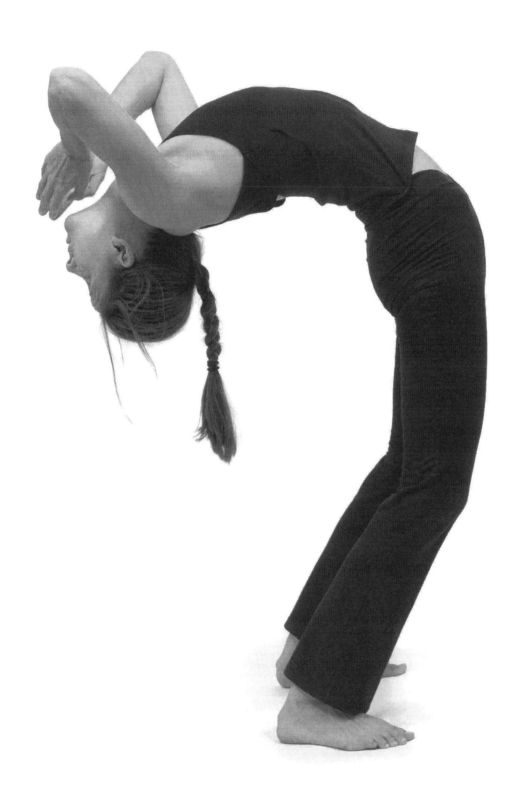

URDHVA DHANURASANA ... continued

Then, walk the hands as close to the feet as possible, tilting the head back and looking toward the feet. Shift the weight of the torso forward over the feet, and press into the soles of the feet. Inhale, standing up, keeping the torso arched back and raising the head last.

Exhale, drop the head as you arch the spine back. Slowly lower the arms down to the floor over the head until the palms of the hands press into the floor, shoulder width of apart.

Inhale, shift the weight forward again over the feet and stand up. Exhale, slowly drop back. Inhale, shift the weight of the hips forward and stand up a third time.

Step the feet together. Inhale, raise the arms above the head and look up to the thumbs. Exhale fold forward into Uttanasana. Inhale, raise the head until the spine and arms straighten, keeping the finger tips in contact with the floor. Press the palms of the hands into the floor, keeping the head lifted, and hop back into Chaturanga Dandasana. Inhale, Urdhva Mukha Shvanasana. Exhale, Adho Mukha Shvanasana.

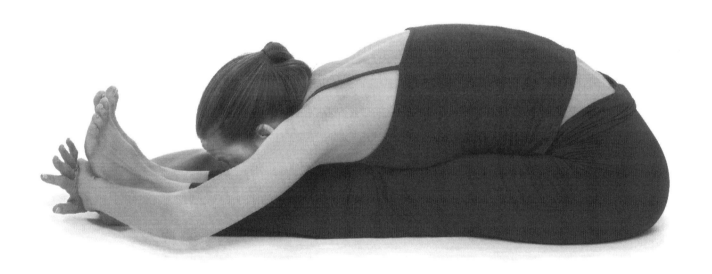

PASCHIMOTTANASANA

Hop forward through the arms into a seated position.
Straighten the legs, flex the feet and press the thighs into
the floor. Reach forward around the feet and take hold of
the left wrist with the right hand. Inhale and raise the head
until the arms and spine straighten while keeping the hands
clasped around the feet. Exhale, pulling the ribcage forward
and down until the torso presses against the legs. Reach
the chin forward and look towards the feet—pada drishti.
Remain here for ten deep breaths.

Sit up, press the palms of the hands into the floor on either
side of the hips. Lift the legs and cross the feet, swinging
back into Chaturanga Dandasana. Inhale, Urdhva Mukha
Shvanasana. Exhale, Adho Mukha Shvanasana.

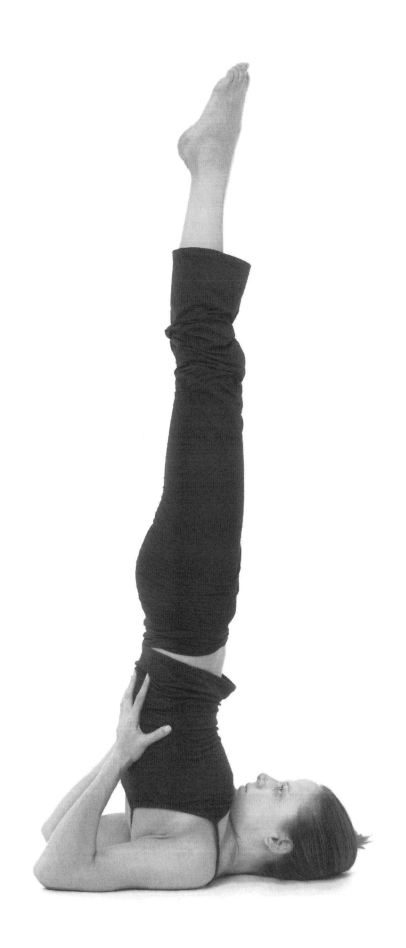

ASHTANGA YOGA

SARVANGASANA

Hop through the arms and lie down on the back. Extend the arms down to the sides, with the palms of the hands facing down and the legs together. Exhale and raise the legs, keeping them straight. Inhale, reach the feet over the head, lift the hips and then extend the feet up to the sky. Shifting the weight of the body into the back of the head and shoulders, bring the legs in line with the spine. Then, bend the elbows, keeping them shoulder width apart, and place the palms of the hands on the back of the ribcage with the fingers pointing up. Point the toes. Keep the chin slightly lifted, shrug the shoulders and draw the shoulder blades towards each other so that the back of the neck does not press into the floor. To adjust the shoulders, feel free to lower the feet down to the floor over the head before raising them back up into Sarvangasana. Allow the chin to press against the sternum and lower the hands down the ribcage towards the floor in order to raise the feet higher up to the sky. Press the legs together gently, soften the eyes and look towards the nose—nasa drishti. Remain in Sarvangasana for ten deep breaths.

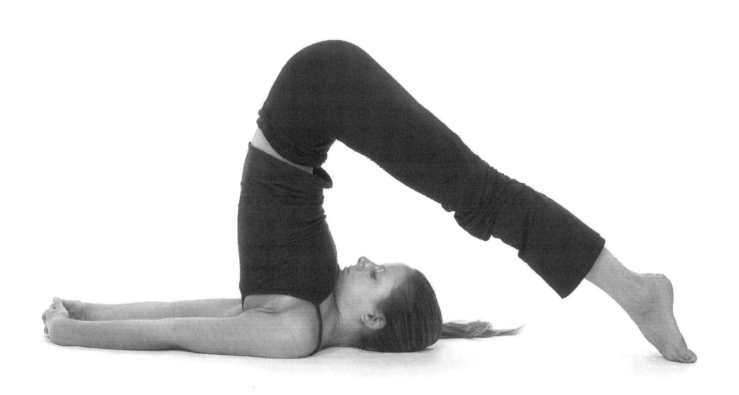

HALASANA

Exhale, lower the legs down to the floor, keeping them straight and together. Straighten the arms, press them into the floor and interlace the fingers. Draw the shoulder blades together and keep the chin level so that the back of the neck does not press into the floor. Point the toes and extend the feet away from the head on the floor. Press the tops of the toes into the floor and slightly raise the sit bones. Look toward the tip of the nose—nasa drishti—and breathe deeply for five breaths.

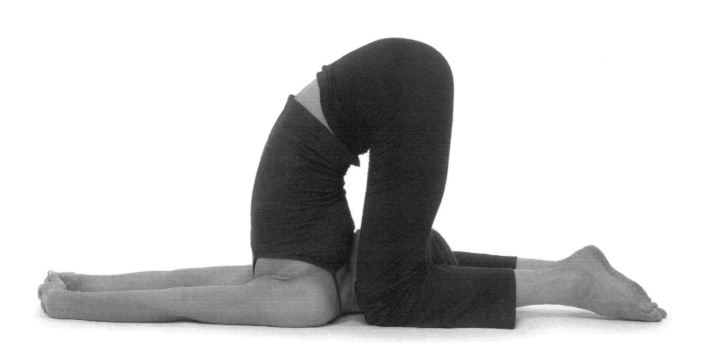

KARNAPIDASANA

Exhale, bend the knees and place them on the floor on either side of the head. Keep the toes pointed and the outsides of the big toes touching. Press the knees gently against the ears. Keep the fingers interlaced and the arms pressing into the floor away from the back. Look toward the tip of the nose— nasa drishti—and breathe deeply for five breaths.

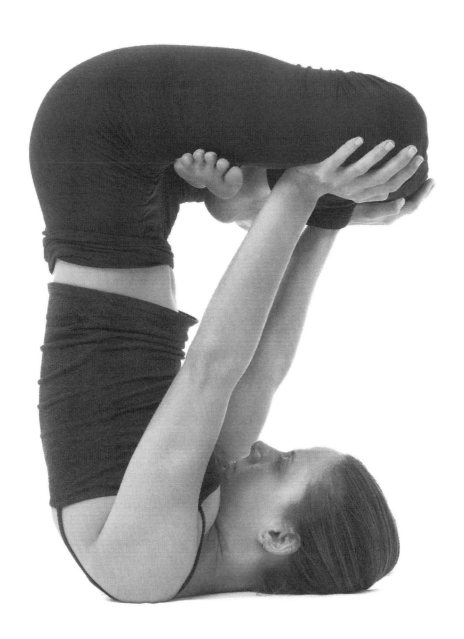

URDHVA PADMASANA

Raise the legs back into Sarvangasana. Bend the right leg and place the outside of the right foot against the left thigh, just above the left hip. Then bend the left leg and place the outside of the left foot against the right thigh, just above the right hip. Lower the knees, keeping the spine straight and the hips lifted, until the legs are parallel to the floor. Balance on the back of the head and shoulders and place the palms of the hands on the inside of the knees, keeping the arms straight. Press the knees against the hands and allow the top of the upper arm bone to press into the floor. Keep the chin level and rest the sternum against the chin. Look toward the tip of the nose—nasa drishti—and take five deep breaths.

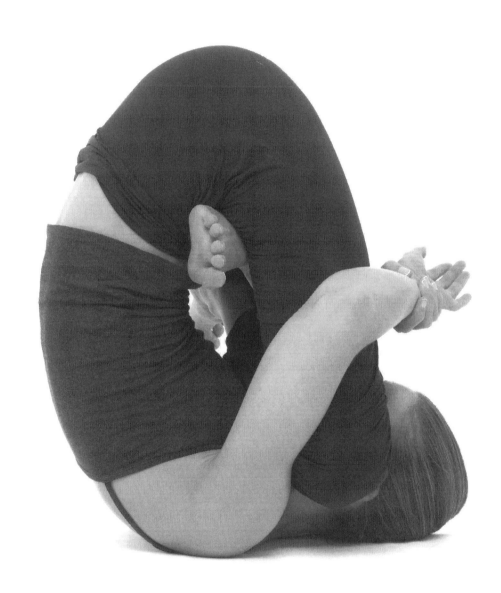

PINDASANA

Keeping the legs folded in Padmasana, lower the knees down to either side of the head and wrap the arms around the legs. Take hold of the left wrist with the right hand and draw the legs in towards the chest. Stay balanced on the back of the head and shoulders. Look softly toward the tip of the nose—nasa drishti—and take five deep breathes in Pindasana.

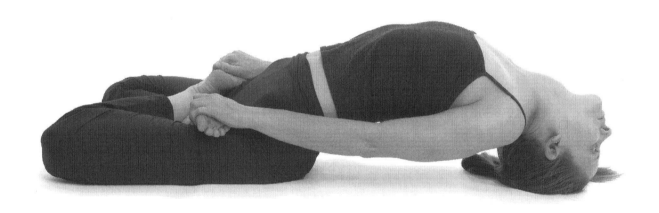

MATSYASANA

Extend the arms on the floor away from the head. Slowly lower the hips to the floor, keeping the legs folded in Padamasana. Then, lower the knees to the floor. Press the elbows into the floor and raise the rib cage, allowing the head to drop back. Place the top of the head on the floor, retaining a deep arch in the upper spine. Then, lift the arms and reach towards the feet, taking hold of left foot with the right hand and the right foot with the left hand. Use the arms to draw the top of the head closer to the hips on the floor. Look up into the forehead—ajna drishti—and remain in Matsyasana for five deep breaths.

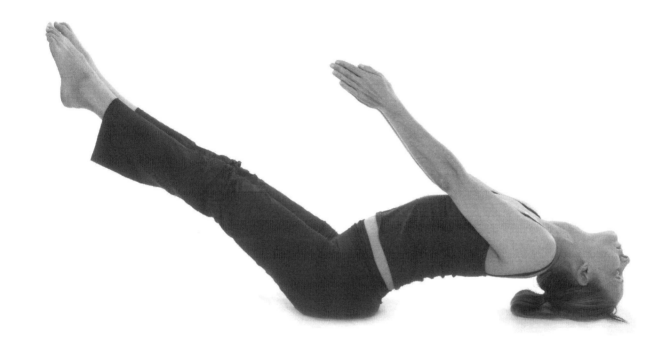

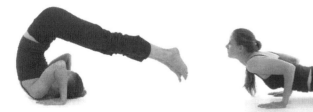 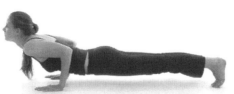 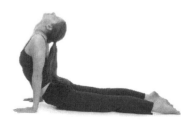

UTTANA PADASANA

Keep the top of the head on the floor and the ribcage lifted. Release the grip of the hands on the feet. Raise the knees and extend the legs 45 degrees off the floor. Draw the legs towards each other and point the toes. Raise the arms and straighten them, pressing the palms of the hands together. Extend the arms out over the torso, parallel to the legs. Look up into the forehead and take five deep breathes.

Keeping the legs raised, lower the arms and press the elbows into the floor on either side of the torso. Lift the ribcage until the head lifts up off of the floor, draw the chin in towards the chest and place the ribcage and back of the head on the floor. Exhale and swing the legs over the head, through Chakrasana into Chaturanga Dandasana. Inhale, Urdhva Mukha Shvansana. Exhale, Adho Mukha Shvanasana.

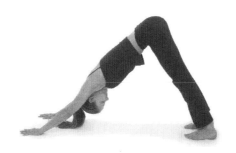

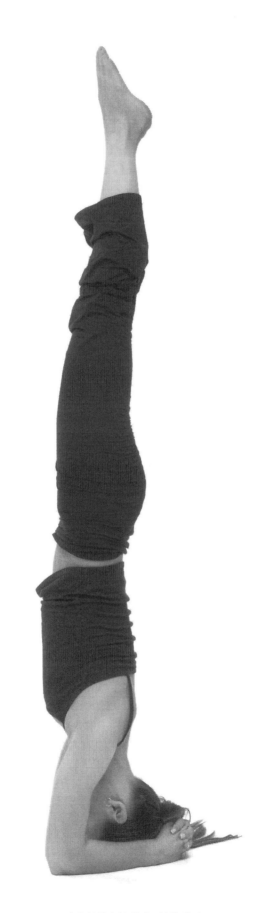

ASHTANGA YOGA

SHIRSHASANA A

Lower the knees down to the floor from Adho Mukha
Shvansana. Interlace the fingers and place the forearms on
the floor with the elbows shoulder width apart. Place the top
of the head on the floor, with the back of the head resting
against the palms of the hands. Raise the hips above the head
by pressing the toes and elbows into the floor and bringing the
legs together and straightening them. On the inhaling breath,
raise the legs, keeping them straight above the head in line
with the torso. Keep the weight of the body off of the top the
head by pressing the forearms into the floor. Point the toes,
look at the nose—nasa drishti—and balance in Shirshasana for
ten deep breaths.

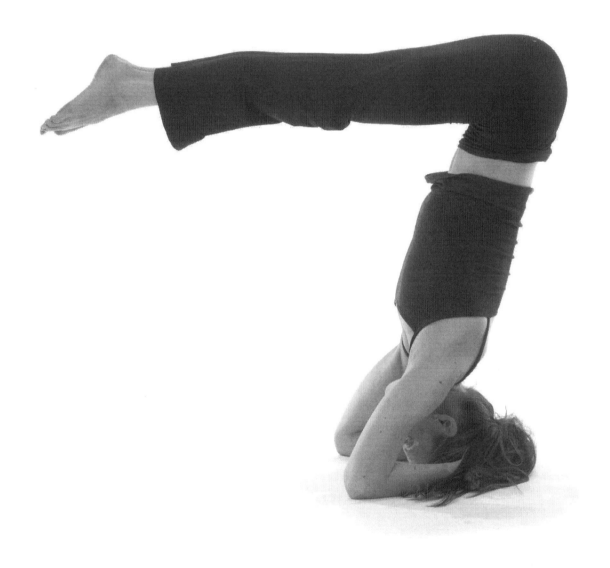

SHIRSHASANA B

Exhale and draw the hips back slightly while lowering the legs and keeping them straight until they are parallel to the floor. Point the toes and look to the nose—nasa drishti. Take five deep breaths in this position.

Inhale and raise the legs back up into Shirshasana. Exhale, lower the feet all the way down to the floor, keeping the legs straight and toes pointed.

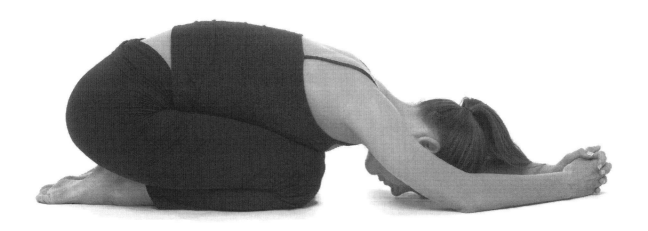

BALASANA

When, coming down from Shirshasana, as the top of the toes touch the floor, begin bending the knees and lowering them to the floor. Keep the feet and knees together and the head in contact with the floor. Then, lower the hips down onto the heels and allow the weight of the head to roll onto the forehead. Keep the arms extended out in front of you or extend them down to either side of the body with the palms of the hands facing up. Look softly toward the tip of the nose—nasa drishti. Breath deeply for five breaths.

Then, on the exhale, place the palms of the hands on the floor on either side of the knees and hop back into Chaturanga Dandasana. Inhale, Urdhva Mukha Shvanasana. Exhale, Adho Mukha Shvanasana.

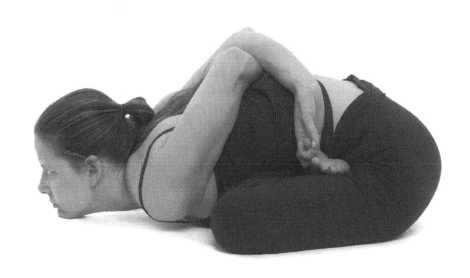

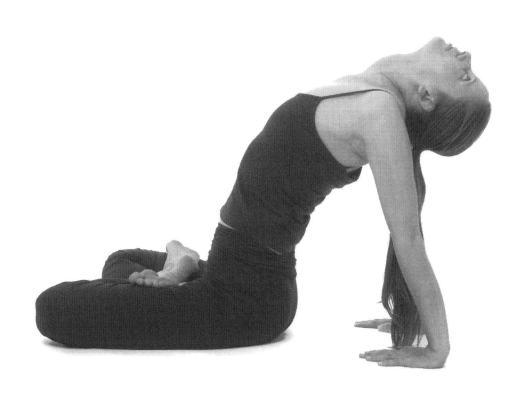

YOGAMUDRA

Hop through the arms into a seated position, with the legs together and extended out in front of you. Bend the right leg and place the top of the right foot on the top of the left thigh, close to the left hip. Bend the left leg and place the top of the left foot on top of the right inner thigh, close to the top of the right hip. Reach the right arm behind the back and take hold of the right big toe with the first two fingers and thumb of the right hand. Reach the left arm behind the back and take hold of the left big toe, with the first two fingers and thumb of the left hand. Fold forward, reaching the chin forward and placing the chin on the floor. Look toward the nose—nasa drishti.

Breathe deeply for five deep breaths.

Inhale, raise the torso and release the arms. Reach the arms back behind you, tilt the head back and place the palms of the hands on the floor shoulder width apart with the finger tips pointing forward.

Press into the hands and extend the ribcage forward and up in order to open the ribcage. Arch the spine back deeply. Look up to the forehead—ajna drishti. Breathe deeply for five breaths.

Inhale back up to sitting, by extending the ribcage forward and lowering the chin last.

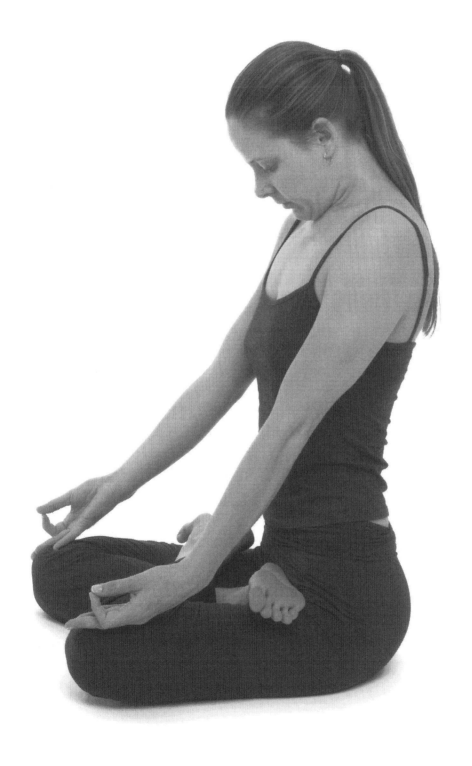

PADMASANA

Keeping the arms straight, rotate them externally and place the back of the hands on the knees. Touch the tips of the thumbs to the tips of the first fingers, and straighten and point the remaining three fingers on both hands away from the wrists. Lift the ribcage and lower the chin down onto the top of the sternum. Contract the muscles in the pelvic floor (Mula Bandha) and draw the navel back to the spine. Look toward the tip of the nose—nasa drishti. Breathe deeply for 25 breaths. Spread the ribcage evenly in all directions on the inhale, and keep the chin in contact with the sternum throughout the cycle of the breath.

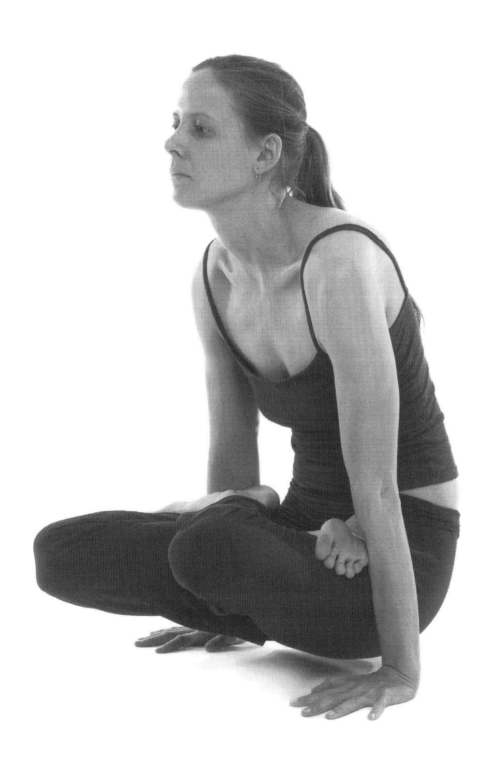

UTH PLUTIHI

Raise the chin so that it is parallel to the floor, placing the palms of the hands on the floor on either side of the hips shoulder width apart. Press into the hands with straight arms and lift the hips and knees off of the floor. Look toward the nose and take 10 deep breaths.

Lower the hips and knees back down to the floor, and swing back into Chaturanga Dandasana on the exhaling breath. Inhale, Urdhva Mukha Shvanasana. Exhale, Adho Mukha Shvanasana.

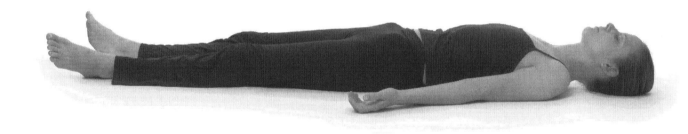

SHAVASANA

Hop through the arms, straighten the legs out in front of you and lie down on the back. Extend the arms down to the sides of the torso with the palms facing up. Relax the legs and allow them to rotate externally. Close the eyes, and release the weight of the body into the floor. Relax in Shavasana for five to ten minutes

Lying on the back on the ground like a corpse is Shavasana. It removes fatigue and gives rest to the mind.

Hatha Yoga Pradipika - Chapter 1, Verse 32

Made in the USA
San Bernardino, CA
17 June 2014